Theory and practice in human services

Neil Thompson

Open University Press
Maidenhead

Open University Press
McGraw-Hill Education
McGraw-Hill House
Shoppenhangers Road
Maidenhead
Berkshire
SL6 2QL

email: enquiries@openup.co.uk
world wide web: www.openup.co.uk

First published in 1995 as *Theory and Practice in Health and Social Welfare*
Reprinted in 1995, 1996 and 1998

First published in this edition 2000
Reprinted 2001, 2003

A catalogue record of this book is available from the British Library

ISBN 0 335 20425 2 (pbk) 0 335 20426 0 (hbk)

Library of Congress Cataloging-in-Publication Data
Thompson, Neil. 1955–
Theory and practice in human services / Neil Thompson.
p. cm.
Rev. ed. of: Theory and practice in health and social welfare.
1995
Includes bibliographical references (p.) and index.
ISBN 0–335–20426–0 (HB). ISBN 0–335–20425–2 (PB)
1. Social service—Research. 2. Human services—Research.
3. Social service—Philosophy. 4. Human services—Philosophy.
5. Social work education. I. Thompson, Neil 1955– Theory and practice in health and social welfare. II. Title.
HV11.T52 2000
361.007–dc21 99–37620 CIP

Typeset by Type Study, Scarborough
Printed and bound in Great Britain by Marston Book Services Limited, Oxford

For Colin

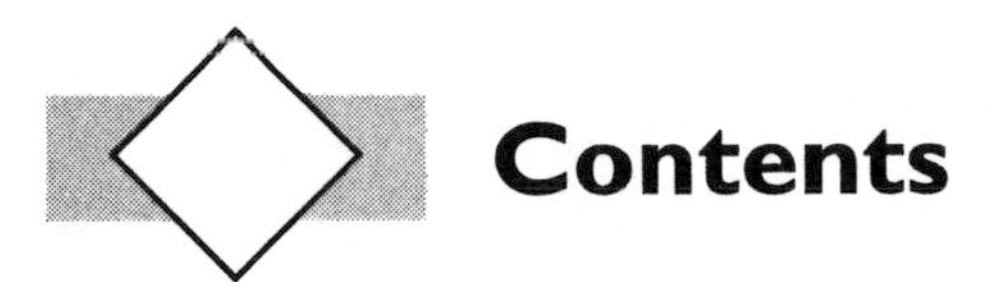

Contents

Preface to the first edition (then entitled *Theory and Practice in Health and Social Welfare)* xi

Preface to the second edition xiii

Acknowledgements xv

Introduction 1

1 **Theory and practice: thinking and doing** 4

Chapter overview 4

Introduction 4

Learning from experience 5

Professionalism 7

Anti-discriminatory practice 10

Power, ideology and values 14

Power 14

Ideology 15

Values 16

The value of research 17

Conclusion 18

Food for thought 19

2 **What is theory?** 21

Chapter overview 21

Introduction 21

Frameworks of understanding 22

Stage 1: The problematic 22

Stage 2: The model 22

Stage 3: Theories 23

Types and levels of theory 25

The importance of theory 30

Anti-discriminatory practice 31

The fallacy of theoryless practice 32
Evaluation 33
Continuous professional development 34
Professional accountability 35
Inappropriate responses 35
The bias of theory 36
Evaluating theories 38
Reductionism 38
Essentialism 38
Reification 38
Teleology 39
The mystique of theory 39
Conclusion 41
Food for thought 42

3 **Science and research** 43
Chapter overview 43
Introduction 43
The critique of positivism 44
Universal laws 45
Objectivity 45
Value-free science 46
Empirical research 48
The distinctiveness of social science 49
Alternatives to positivism 50
Hermeneutical science 51
Critical theory 52
Postmodernism 53
The role of research 53
Types of research 55
Research criteria 57
Validity 57
Reliability 57
Rigour 58
Objectivity 58
Explanatory power 58
The limitations of research 59
Conclusion: research-minded practice 60
Food for thought 62

The philosophical basis 63
Chapter overview 63
Introduction 63
What is philosophy? 64
Beyond eclecticism 67
Dialectical reason 68

Postmodernism 70
Fragmentation 70
Logocentrism 71
Différance 71
Affirmation of diversity 72
Existentialism 72
Lived experience 79
Existentialist practice 80
Conclusion 81
Food for thought 83

Narrowing the gap 84
Chapter overview 84
Introduction 84
Why does a gap exist? 85
Developing reflective practice 87
Beyond reflection 91
Integrating theory and practice 93
Strategies for integration 94
Using cycles of learning 95
Going beyond practice wisdom 95
Going beyond theoryless practice 96
Going beyond common sense 97
Developing research-minded practice 98
Going beyond elitism and anti-intellectualism 99
Using the critical incident technique 100
Developing a group approach 101
Promoting continuous professional development 102
Developing interprofessional learning 103
Using mentoring 104
Problematizing 104
Using enquiry and action learning (EAL) 105
Balancing challenge and support 106
Developing staff care 106
Conclusion 107
Food for thought 108

6 **Education and training: human resource development** 109
Chapter overview 109
Introduction 109
Education or training? 110
Knowledge, skills and values 112
Competence-based training: for and against 118
Person-centred learning 122
Conclusion 127
Food for thought 128

The adventure of theory 129
Chapter overview 129
Introduction 129
The organizational context 130
Continuous professional development 133
The practitioner as theorist 135
Dealing with uncertainty 138
Making it happen 140
Conclusion 144
Food for thought 145

Glossary 146

References 152

Index 161

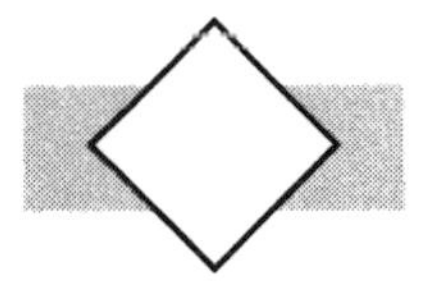

Preface to the first edition

A long-established task of professional education in health care and social work is to facilitate the integration of theory and practice, to help make professional practice an *informed* practice. The process of applying theory to practice is one which is strongly encouraged and highly valued, in certain quarters at least. It remains, however, a relatively poorly understood process and continues to confuse and bewilder students and practitioners alike – and, of course, educationalists are not necessarily *au fait* with the subleties and intricacies of this multi-layered area. Although much has been written on this topic, a clear and comprehensive account of the process remains elusive.

This text is not presented as the answer to this particular prayer, but it does have an important play in clarifying and demystifying many aspects of the complex interweavings of theory and practice. It will certainly not answer all the questions, but it should equip us to address these questions more fully and in a more informed way. In this way, it offers a basis from which to develop a clearer grasp of theory–practice integration, to understand why it is so important and to feel more confident in tackling some of the difficulties involved in developing a practice grounded in relevant theory and values.

Readers looking for a simple answer to the question of applying theory to practice will no doubt be disappointed, but readers willing to get to grips with a set of very demanding and thorny issues will, I hope, gain a great deal of help and encouragement to support them in this endeavour.

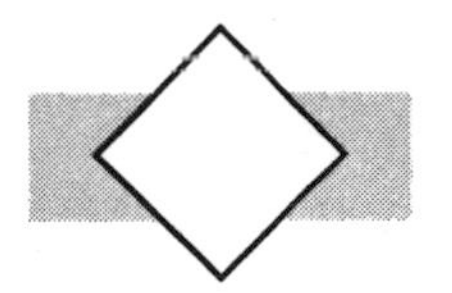

Preface to the second edition

In the five years since the first edition of this book was published, both theory and practice have continued to move on and evolve. There have been new developments in policy and practice and, of course many more theoretical treatises in books and journals as well as a steady stream of research reports. The whole area remains a vibrant one, with work continuing at several levels within and across disciplines. Of course, this new edition will not attempt to incorporate all such changes, as that would clearly be a hopelessly ambitious task. Rather, my more modest aim is to provide a much more limited exploration of developments in the relationship between theory and practice.

The basic challenge remains pretty much the same as it was five years ago: to seek a better understanding of the factors which facilitate the optimal integration of theory and practice and those which hinder the process, with a view to developing a basis for the enhancement of both theory and practice. While myths about the role and value of theory, research and formal knowledge continue to hold sway in so many settings, the development of high-quality practice will be hampered unnecessarily. It is to be hoped, then, that this edition will build on the success of the first in helping people appreciate both the complexities of theory and practice *and* the need to find ways of maximizing the benefits of a theoretically informed approach to practice.

Feedback on the first edition has, I am pleased to say, been very positive indeed. It is very rewarding to note that many people have found my exploration of these complex issues helpful and illuminating. I hope this edition will prove similarly helpful. However, it remains the case that the book is not intended to provide definitive answers or step-by-step sets of instructions to follow. Indeed, it is a central premise of the book that theory can provide part of the 'raw material' from which practice responses can be fashioned, but cannot realistically be expected to provide 'off-the-peg' solutions. This book too comes into that category.

The focus of this edition has been widened in the sense that reference is made to the human services more broadly (social work and social care; nursing and health care; probation and community justice; youth and community work; counselling, advocacy and advice work; and so on) rather than the narrower field of 'health and social welfare'. This widening of readership is in response to the fact that so many people have pointed out to me that most of the points I made in the first edition in relation to nursing and/or social work could be seen to apply more broadly to the human services in general. Perhaps inevitably, though, it remains the case that my own background in social work is likely to have a bearing on the way the subject matter is treated. In keeping with the spirit of reflective practice, it is apt that practitioners and students across the various disciplines should face the challenge of taking the points made in this book and adapting them to their own professional arena, rather than look for direct 'answers' in this text.

There continue to be no easy answers, but there remain a number of avenues that can be explored to make progress in trying to bridge the traditional gap between theory and practice so that the two fields can inform each other and both gain from the interaction.

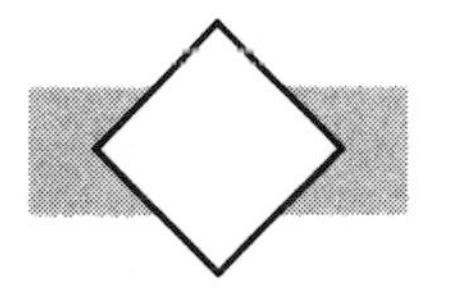

Acknowledgements

Many people played an important supporting role in developing the first edition of this book. In particular, I benefited from the involvement of Irene Thompson and Graham Thompson of the University of Wales, Bangor; Ann Smith and Jacqui Russell of the University of Northumbria; Colin Richardson, Fellow of Keele University; John Bates of North East Wales Institute of Higher Education; and Clive Curtis of Cheshire County Council.

Joyce Thompson did an excellent job of typing the manuscript, and the artwork on which the front cover is based is due to the artistic skills of Jen Randles. Susan Thompson was, as always, unstinting in her moral, practical and intellectual support.

For this second edition I continue to be grateful to those who played a significant part in the development of the original text. In addition I am very grateful to the very many people who have shared their views with me on the use of theory in practice and the development of reflective practice. This includes a wide range of students, practitioners and educators in various settings. They have all played at least a small part in providing the stimulus for the continuing development of my thinking on these important themes, and for that I am extremely grateful.

The author and publishers would like to acknowledge the kind permission of the Open University to reproduce Figure 2.1, taken from summer school teaching materials and Whiting and Birch to reproduce Figure 2.2, taken from Sibeon (1990).

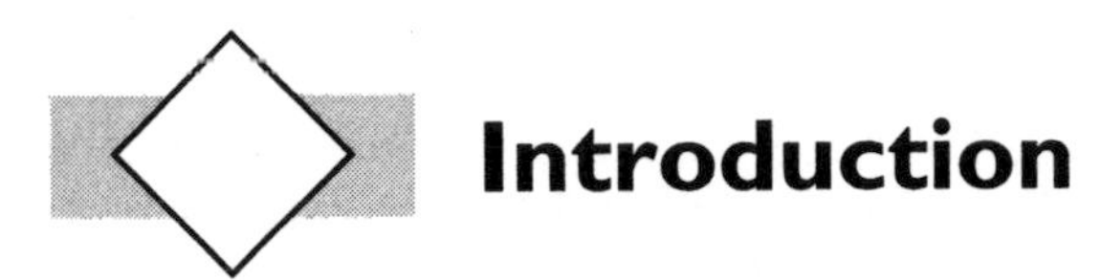

Introduction

Within social work, nursing and the other human services, phrases like 'applying theory to practice' or 'integrating theory and practice' are often used, especially where issues of education, training and staff development are high on the agenda. But what do these mean? What does the process of relating theory to practice actually involve? What is it that takes place? And is it necessarily a good thing? These are some of the key questions that underpin this book. Indeed, this book could be seen as an attempt to unravel some of the complexities associated with these and related questions.

The existence and use of a theory base or body of formal knowledge are strongly associated with the notion of 'professionalism' – and the occupational credibility that professional status can be seen to bestow. There are, therefore, powerful reasons why theory is seen as being of value in terms of status and respect. However, if these reasons were the only ones, the use of theory would be a hollow sham, a false pretence. In this book, I shall therefore be presenting a range of other arguments as to why a sound and appropriate theory base is important. Indeed, I shall argue that this is not only important, but is, in fact, essential for maximizing the potential effectiveness of human services practice.

These arguments will be explained in more detail in each of the chapters that follow. However, the underlying theme or principle on which the book is based is that theory is a primary part of *informed* practice, and that informed practice is necessary to:

- do justice to the complexity of the situations human services workers so frequently encounter;
- avoid assumptions, prejudices and stereotypes that can lead to discrimination and oppression;
- lay the foundations for a *developmental* approach, one which permits and facilitates continuous personal and professional development;
- ensure a high level of motivation, challenge and commitment.

Despite the value of making use of theory in practice, there are, however, two sets of factors that stand in the way of this. On the one hand, many practitioners reject theory and prefer to adopt what they see as a pragmatic or 'common sense' approach. On the other hand, much theoretical knowledge has traditionally been expressed in impenetrable highbrow terms, making the material appear elitist and inaccessible, and therefore of little use to practitioners. This is therefore a book about building bridges, or at least one major bridge – that between theory and practice, thinking and doing. This is to be achieved by challenging the rejection of theory through showing the problems a supposedly non-theoretical approach leads to, and by seeking to dispel much of the mystique and elitism that surrounds the world of theory.

In one way, of course, this book reflects a significant irony. It is intended as a reflective tool to help practitioners, managers and educationalists get to grips with some of the thorny issues of relating theory to practice, and yet those people who have little or no awareness of the significance of theory are probably the people least likely to read the book. None the less, it is offered as an aid to understanding for those who see the value of tackling these issues as a means of improving practice.

The book is divided into seven chapters, each with its own major theme or focus. However, due to the nature of the subject matter, it is inevitable that there is some overlap between the chapters and a number of recurring themes will be evident. It is to be hoped, then, that the book succeeds in capturing both the diversity of theory and the underlying commonalities.

Chapter 1 examines the role of theory in training, education and professional development. It addresses the question of how adults learn and identifies some of the common obstacles to learning. This chapter also comments on the dangers of relying on 'common sense', a theme to be developed in more detail later.

Chapter 2 poses the fundamental question, 'What is theory?' It examines the role of research and formal knowledge in guiding practice. Similarly, the concept of 'practice wisdom' is introduced and its contribution to professional practice is evaluated. This chapter also considers the absence of race and gender issues in traditional theory, and the ethnocentric and gender biases these absences lead to.

Chapter 3 focuses on the scientific nature of theory. It considers how social science knowledge differs from the natural sciences, and highlights some of the problems associated with applying a natural science model to the helping professions. This chapter also addresses the nature, use and limitations of research, with particular reference to the concept of 'research-minded practice' (Everitt *et al.* 1992).

Chapter 4 builds on some of the themes raised in Chapter 3 by exploring a number of the aspects of the philosophical basis of human services practice. In particular, the role of values is considered in relation to both theory and practice. The problems of combining theories uncritically are identified and existentialism is presented as a valuable philosophical perspective on human services. Due to the complex nature of the subject matter covered here, this chapter is perhaps a little less easy to get to grips with than the others, although efforts have been made to make it 'user-friendly' so that the important issues discussed are not lost in a web of words.

Chapter 5 has as its main theme the task of 'narrowing the gap' between theory and practice. It explores a number of ways in which theory and practice can be successfully and usefully integrated. A central concept in this chapter is that of 'reflective practice', and this is proposed as an important link in the chain of relating theory to practice.

Chapter 6 revisits some of the issues raised in Chapter 1 concerning adult learning and professional development. In particular, it examines the tension between education and training and considers the respective contributions each can make. This chapter also explores competence-based training and weighs up the main advantages and disadvantages of such an approach.

Chapter 7 discusses the 'adventure of theory', the benefits that can be obtained from developing a practice based on relevant theory and values. It tries to give a flavour of the motivation, commitment and job satisfaction that can be gained from adopting an approach to practice informed by theory. This chapter also explores the organizational context in terms of organizational culture. Chapter 7 is also the concluding chapter, and it summarizes the arguments presented and the issues covered. It draws out the lessons that can be learned and the conclusions that can be drawn.

Theory and practice: thinking and doing

Chapter overview

- How does thinking influence doing?
- What is involved in the process of learning?
- What is professionalism?
- What is anti-discriminatory practice?
- Why is research important?

Introduction

The relationship between theory and practice can be seen as a direct parallel with that between thinking and doing. It hinges on the question: 'How do knowledge and thought influence or inform our actions?' In a sense, the whole book is concerned with this question as there is no simple or straightforward answer. However, the particular focus within this opening chapter is on the processes of learning and related issues, and the ways in which such processes apply to the integration of theory and practice.

I shall begin by introducing a model of learning that helps to cast some light on what happens when theory is applied to practice. This sets the scene for a discussion of professionalism and the key concept of a professional knowledge base, as reflected in the identified requirements of bodies responsible for overseeing education and training provision (for example, CCETSW 1991; UKCC 1986).

Another key aspect of this chapter is the consideration of issues of anti-discriminatory practice and the promotion of equality. In particular, the role of power, ideology and values in influencing both theory and practice is explored. And, finally, the value of research is considered, and the need for reflective practice is emphasized.

In many ways, this is a 'foundation' chapter in so far as it introduces a number of themes and issues which will be revisited later in the text. In this respect, the task of this chapter is to 'set the scene' for the remainder of the book by highlighting the complexities of the subject matter to be covered while beginning to develop a framework for helping to make sense of them.

Learning from experience

The work of David Kolb and associated theorists (Kolb *et al.* 1979; Kolb and Fry 1975; Kolb 1984) has had a major influence on our understanding of educational processes and the significance of these for training and development. In particular, Kolb's notion of the 'learning cycle' has become well established as a tool for understanding adult learning. Kolb's ideas are summarized here as they can be seen as a useful introduction to the idea of learning as an active process. It should be noted, however, that the question of adult learning is a complex one and Kolb's learning cycle should not be seen as a definitive statement on the subject.

The cycle involves four stages. The first is that of *concrete experience*. This can refer to experiences specifically geared towards learning – reading, attending a training course and so on – or, more broadly, one's life experience in general. This immediately introduces two key underpinnings of Kolb's model of learning. First, it can be seen that learning is based on life experience rather than just formal opportunities for learning. Second, this is a positive and optimistic model of learning – opportunities for learning abound.

However, concrete experience in itself is not enough to promote learning, and this is where the second stage comes in, that of *reflective observation*. This involves reflecting on the experience and considering its significance. In short, we cannot learn from experience unless we actually think about that experience, and thereby make sense of it.

This, in turn, sets the scene for the third stage, that of *abstract conceptualization*. Reflective observation opens the door for a broader and deeper consideration of the issues arising from one's experience. The experience can be linked to other experiences, beliefs and attitudes and thus integrated into one's overall life experience. This entails considering the implications of the concrete experience and evaluating its relevance and validity. Such conceptualizing frequently entails forming a hypothesis or 'working model' of the situation (Thompson *et al.* 1994b: 38). The notion of 'hypothesis formation' is an important one, and one to which we shall return in Chapter 7 when Kelly's (1955) theory of constructive alternativism is discussed.

The fourth stage of the cycle is that of *active experimentation*. This is the point at which the new learning is tried out in practice, when learning at an abstract level is translated into the concrete reality of practice. Although this now completes the cycle, this is not the end of the story, as the fourth stage now becomes the first stage (concrete experience) of a new cycle of learning. And so the process continues.

Implicit within this model is a perspective on the relationship between theory and practice. This perspective can be described in terms of the following propositions:

1. Learning does not happen automatically as a result of experience. Our experience has to be 'processed' (reflected upon, related to previous learning and applied to practice) in order for learning to take place. This 'processing' is, in effect, part of relating theory to practice.
2. In order to make sense of our experience, we have to integrate it within a framework of pre-existing concepts – we have to make it part of our own theory base. (This is a point to which I shall return in Chapter 2.) In this way, we are 'applying practice to theory', using our new experience to test and extend our theoretical understanding of the world.
3. Full learning only takes place when the cycle is completed, when learning is put into practice. If we only go as far as stage 3 and do not engage in 'active experimentation', we may have acquired knowledge, but we will not have *learned*. Acquiring knowledge is only part of the process of learning.
4. Each of us is responsible for our own learning. Learning is an active and self-directed process and so, ultimately, no one can do our learning for us. Others can facilitate or encourage our learning but no one can make us learn – that is a matter that lies in our own hands. Similarly, relating theory to practice must be a matter for which we each take responsibility – to translate knowledge into action and complete the learning cycle.

Kolb's approach to learning has much in common with the notion of 'reflective practice' as developed by theorists such as Schön (1983), Boud *et al.* (1985) and Powell (1989a). Coutts-Jarman (1993) refers us to the earlier work of Dewey, whose ideas have proven very influential with regard to our understanding of reflective practice:

> Dewey (1933) first made a distinction between routine and reflective human action. He stated that routine action is action guided by impulse, tradition and authority. The routine practitioner takes the everyday realities of practice for granted, e.g. its concepts, problems and goals, and concentrates on discovering the more effective and efficient means of solving the problem. He then defined reflective action as '. . . active, persistent and

> careful consideration of any belief or supposed knowledge in the light of the grounds that support it and the further consequences to which it leads'.
>
> (Coutts-Jarman 1993: 78)

This is similar to what Hopkins (1986) refers to as 'informed and sensitive practice'. Implicit within the notion is the belief in the greater value of a practice based on thought and reflection than one based on routine and assumption. Indeed, this belief in the greater value of reflective practice will become a recurring theme in the chapters that follow.

Before moving on, it is perhaps worth re-emphasizing point 4 above, namely the axiom that the learner is responsible for his or her own learning. This is a point, the significance of which is not always fully appreciated. As Boud and Walker (1990: 62) comment:

> There is potential for learning in every situation and it is up to the learner to realise this potential. It is the learner's interaction with the learning milieu which creates the particular learning experience. While facilitators, and others, can create the milieu, it is the learner who creates the experience.

The same logic can be applied to the use of theory in practice. That is, day-to-day practice provides a milieu in which 'thinking' and 'doing' are in constant interaction. This provides opportunities for learning (doing enhances thinking) but also creates opportunities for using theoretical and other knowledge as a framework for understanding and a guide to action (thinking enhances doing). But, as Boud and Walker imply, the milieu provides opportunities but these opportunities do not, of themselves, produce learning. Similarly, opportunities for putting theory into practice do not automatically produce theory-based practice. Practitioners have a responsibility for converting those opportunities into an enhanced level of practice.

In short, both learning and relating theory to practice are active processes – they will not happen unless the individual concerned takes some degree of initiative and makes some commitment to taking the process forward. This is a feature of 'reflective practice', a concept I shall discuss in more detail in Chapter 5.

Professionalism

One of the recognized hallmarks of a profession is an underlying knowledge base, a body of specialist knowledge which acts as the basis of professional expertise (Sibeon 1991). In attempting to achieve professional status within the human services, both nursing and social work have been keen to demonstrate not only an underpinning

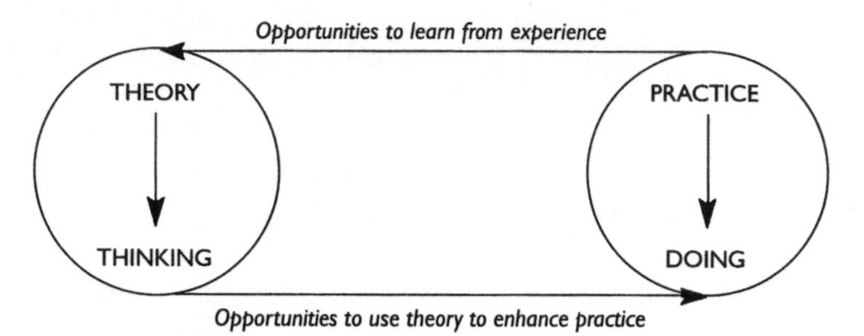

Figure 1.1 Thinking and doing

knowledge base but, more specifically, a *distinctive* knowledge base. This is particularly the case with nursing, due in no small part to the desire to establish it as a profession allied to, but also *distinct from*, the medical profession. For example, Parker and Creasia (1991: 5) seem keen to present nursing as a 'unique body of knowledge', and this seems to reflect a wider anxiety to establish nursing as a theoretical endeavour in its own right.

This drive towards a distinctive theory base is not so evident in social work and social care, although this is not to say that it does not exist. This difference between the two professional groups can be explained, partly at least, by reference to two factors:

1. Nursing is closely associated with medicine, both historically and practically. The impetus to develop a distinctive theory base can be linked to a desire to develop a professional identity separate from the more powerful, and more firmly established, profession of medicine. Social work, by contrast, is not so closely associated with medicine, and so the need to be seen as separate has not been so acutely felt.
2. Social work can be seen to have a more ambivalent attitude towards the value of adopting a 'professional' approach to social problems, influenced by radical social work with its emphasis on the political roots of so many of the problems experienced by social work clients (Corrigan and Leonard 1978; Brake and Bailey 1980; Thompson 1992a). This mistrust of 'professionalism' has a number of effects, including a tendency to devalue theory. Preston-Shoot and Agass (1990: 5) argue that:

   > Social workers have an ambivalent relationship with theory. Uncertain of its relevance, social workers lack an adequate theoretical and conceptual base for purposeful practice. They are often unable to articulate the skills and knowledge which guide their practice, or the specific forms of intervention or practice theory they are applying to their work . . . Theorising is abandoned to academics.

On both counts, then, theory is located within the broader context of aspirations to professionalism. Hugman (1991) comments on the absence of 'a clearly demarcated scientific knowledge base' as a barrier to full professional status, relegating social work and nursing to the 'semi-professions' (Etzioni 1969). This reflects the 'trait' approach to professionalism, an approach which is based on certain defining characteristics or 'traits'. Hugman (1991: 6) is critical of this approach and goes on to argue that: 'The language of professionalism frequently serves to obscure the issue of power'. Indeed, aspiring towards professionalism ('professionalizing' as Sibeon, 1991, puts it) can be seen as a bid for increased power and control. In this sense, professionalism becomes an end in itself (a set of 'perks' for staff), rather than a means to an end (greater benefits for service users as a result of enhanced levels of practice).

However, professionalism can also be presented in a more positive light in terms of:

- a commitment to high standards;
- a set of values and principles to guide practice;
- a degree of autonomous judgement, rather than bureaucratic rule-following;
- acceptance of personal and collective responsibility;
- the use of formal knowledge as part of a process of seeking to maximize effectiveness.

It is, of course, the fifth element which is significant for present purposes, for it is here that the integration of theory and practice can be recognized as an important part of professionalism – a professionalism based on commitment rather than elitism. Organizations responsible for the education and training of staff also place emphasis on the importance of relating theory to practice as a component of professional credibility. For example, the Central Council for Education and Training in Social Work (CCETSW) includes, among its requirements:

> Qualifying social workers must be able to:
> – analyse and evaluate their own and others' personal experience;
> – analyse and clarify concepts and issues;
> – apply knowledge and understanding to practice;
> – use research findings in practice.
>
> (CCETSW 1991: 16)

Clearly, then, the debate about theory–practice integration and the debate about professionalism overlap to a considerable extent. Because of this important set of interconnections, the question of professionalism is one to which we shall return later.

Anti-discriminatory practice

Traditional approaches to the human services take little or no account of issues of discrimination and oppression (Thompson 1998a). Although some aspects of class discrimination have long been recognized (for example, The Black Report concerning class inequalities – Townsend and Davidson 1987), other forms of discrimination have, for the most part, received scant attention. Indeed, it is only since the late 1980s that the issues of sexism, racism and so on have *begun* to make an impact on the social policy agenda in Britain.

Now, however, changes are beginning to be made. These include:

- Legislative changes in which issues of race, culture, gender and so on have been recognized as important factors: The Children Act 1989, The NHS and Community Care Act 1990 and the Criminal Justice Act 1991.
- A growing literature and research base on a range of related topics.
- A commitment to anti-discriminatory practice in vocational education and training (NVQ/SVQ).
- An increasing emphasis on equal opportunities policies and practices and the management of diversity.
- A more prominent and vocal stance on the part of groups of service users, for example the Disabled People's Movement (Oliver 1990; Thompson 1997).
- A growing number of courses and training materials.
- A significant and growing number of people who are interested in, and committed to, the issues.

This is not an exhaustive list, but is sufficient to make the point that change is at least beginning to take place.

An important implication of this that the process of integrating theory and practice must take on board, as a central concern, is a commitment to challenging discrimination and oppression. That is, the task is also one of relating *anti-discriminatory* theory to practice. Indeed, we could say that the primary task is that of using theory to develop anti-discriminatory practice, for as I have argued previously, good practice must be anti-discriminatory practice:

> . . . practice which does not take account of oppression and discrimination cannot be seen as good practice, no matter how high its standards may be in other respects. For example, . . . intervention with a disabled person which fails to recognise the marginalised position of disabled people in society runs the risk of doing the client more of a disservice than a service.
>
> (Thompson 1997: 11)

We cannot, realistically, describe our actions as 'good practice' if such

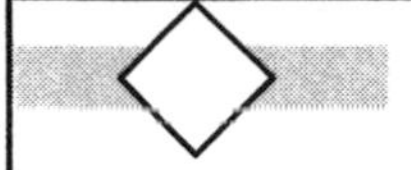

Practice Focus 1.1

Indira Begum was admitted to a nursing home when her family no longer felt able to look after her. At first she seemed to settle well, but soon became very withdrawn and depressed. Her relatives were very impressed with the standard of nursing care in the home and therefore made no connection between the nursing care provided and Indira's deteriorating condition. However, on one particular visit, Indira's daughter noticed an uneaten meal on a tray next to her mother's bed. She was surprised and disappointed to find the meal consisted of traditional western fare, wholly unlike the type of food her mother was accustomed to eating. Further investigation revealed that no allowance had been made for her mother's cultural preferences with regard to food or other aspects of daily living. A picture therefore began to form – a distressing picture in which Indira felt marginalized, alienated and, consequently, devalued.

When the issue was raised with the officer in charge, her response was simple and straightforward. She believed in treating everybody the same – in order to avoid drawing attention to people's differences. Despite the 'good intentions' underlying this 'colour-blind' approach, the actual outcome was a negative and discriminatory one. Despite nursing standards being high in other respects, this lack of sensitivity to ethnic needs had produced a racist outcome.

practice oppresses or discriminates against the people we are working with.

In order to understand how and why this is important, I shall present examples relating to four particular forms of discrimination. Practice Focus illustrations 1.1 to 1.4 relate to racism, sexism, ageism and disablism, respectively. Space does not permit a detailed analysis of these issues and so interested readers are advised to consult Thompson (1997) and/or Thompson (1998a).

In addition to the problems of racism, the discrimination experienced by women – or sexism as it is more commonly known – is also a significant aspect of human services.

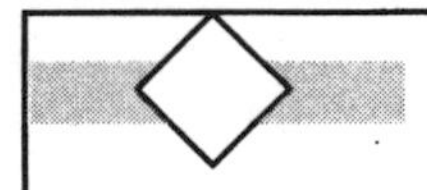

Practice Focus 1.2

Sandra was a student on placement with a multidisciplinary mental health team as part of her professional training. She was very impressed with the high standards of practice in the team and the high level of commitment. However, after returning to college for a day's workshop on gender awareness, she found herself with something of a dilemma.

cont.

Practice Focus 1.2 (*cont.*)

The workshop had drawn her attention to the way in which forms of practice which do not show a sensitivity to gender issues can so easily, and unwittingly, reinforce oppressive and destructive gender stereotypes. The contradiction, for Sandra, was that what had superficially appeared to be good practice was, on closer inspection, potentially very problematic, particularly for women clients. For example, she noticed significant differences in how workers responded to people with depression. Depressed men were being encouraged to overcome their depression by pursuing what she had now come to recognize as typically masculine activities such as work and sport. Depressed women, by contrast, were being encouraged to find a solution in femininity by, for example, pursuing handicrafts, cooking and 'making themselves look pretty'. The possibility that gender role restrictions and sexism were part of the problems leading to depression was one that had not been explored or even considered.

One of the common problems encountered in old age is a tendency to be treated as 'non-persons', as if all humanity is surrendered on reaching a particular age (Thompson 1995a). This is an example of the dehumanization inherent in old age, and also a significant dimension of 'ageism', a form of discrimination which Hughes and Mtezuka (1992: 220) define as: 'the social process through which negative images of and attitudes towards older people, based solely on the characteristics of old age itself, result in discrimination'.

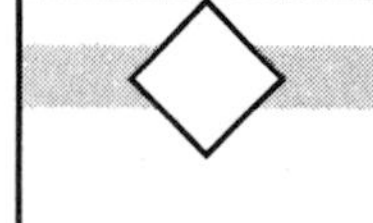

Practice Focus 1.3

Ageism was precisely the problem Rhian encountered when she took up her new post as a day-centre manager. The problem was not one of malice but, rather, one of misguided kindness. Rhian's predecessor had encouraged the staff to 'look after' the users of the centre as best they could. The effect of this had been to create an ethos of dependency in which weaknesses were emphasized, rather than strengths enhanced and reinforced. Consequently, their efforts were counter-productive in so far as they undermined confidence and self-esteem. In effect, this approach was based on ageist stereotypes of frailty and dependency. Rhian therefore set herself the task of developing an ethos of empowerment – to challenge, rather than reinforce, ageism.

Disablism has much in common with ageism in so far as they both focus on weakness and both marginalize groups of people on the basis of stereotypical misconceptions. Disablism involves seeing people with a physical impairment as objects of pity who are not able to participate in mainstream society (Oliver 1990; Oliver and Sapey 1999). Practice Focus 1.4 highlights the underlying problem of disablism – a focus on helping disabled people to 'adjust' to their 'condition':

> The major task of the professional is therefore to adjust the individual to the particular disabling condition. There are two aspects of this: first there is physical adjustment through rehabilitation programmes designed to return the individual to as near normal a state as possible: and second, there is psychological adjustment which helps the individual to come to terms with the physical limitations.
>
> (Oliver 1983: 15)

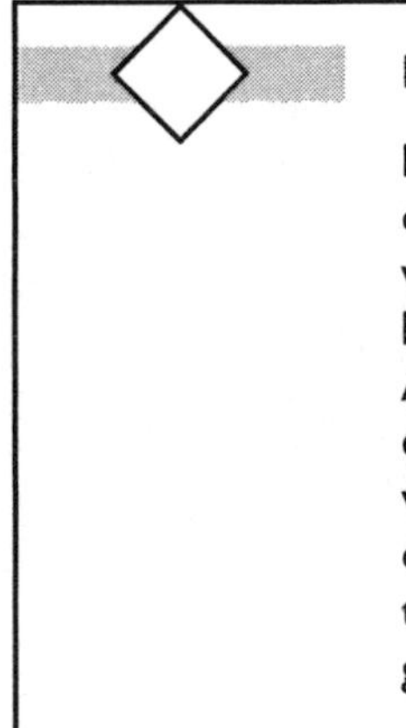

Practice Focus 1.4

Disablism was represented by the actions of a social services department in setting up a working party to plan services for people with disabilities. In order to gain broad representation, staff from the health service and local voluntary agencies were invited to contribute. At one level, this proved to be a success and resulted in a high level of effective multidisciplinary collaboration. However, at another level, the whole exercise proved to be a complete failure. The planning group was only able to provide a professional perspective and took no account of the perspective of disabled people themselves. Consequently, the latter group felt alienated and marginalized – objects rather than subjects.

Oliver is critical of this individualistic model of disability as it overemphasizes the assumed personal costs of disability and under-emphasizes the social and political costs of disability which marginalize disabled people. The problems inherent in this traditional individualistic approach illustrate two important points, indeed two central themes of this book:

1. *Good practice must be anti-discriminatory practice.* An approach to human services work which is not sensitive to issues of discrimination and oppression runs the risk of doing more harm than good and is therefore extremely dangerous.
2. *Practice needs to be based on theory.* A 'common sense' approach would not alert us to the dangers and pitfalls of working in an

individualistic way. Good practice therefore needs to be informed by theoretical understanding.

The four examples given here raise a number of important issues, some of which will be addressed in ensuing chapters. For present purposes, however, it is sufficient to note that issues of discrimination and oppression *must* be central to the debate about theory and practice if we are not to settle for a partial or distorted picture. We should also note that the four areas of discrimination outlined here are not the only ones that need to be taken into consideration. Issues of sexual identity, language, nationality, region and so on are also important considerations. In addition, the question of class – socio-economic position – can be seen to cut across all the forms of oppression and intersect with them. Economic power (or the lack of it) can be a significant factor in relation to oppression at a general level and, more specifically, directly to human services practice. For example, middle-class workers may feel more comfortable in dealing with service users of a similar class background. There is therefore considerable scope for discrimination, intended or otherwise, and so there is a need for sensitivity to issues of class.

It is also important to recognize that discrimination extends far beyond the main categories of class, race, gender and so on. Many groups of people can experience discrimination in certain circumstances. Consider, for example, the following passage from Bevan (1998: 29):

> People who are dying can be seen to be marginalised and discriminated against in many of the ways that other groups defined by age, race, gender and social class are. This exclusion and devaluing may be understood contextually by examining western cultural values which tend to idealise youth, productivity and success.

The concept of discrimination therefore needs to be seen in its widest sense, rather than restricted to the most well-established forms.

Power, ideology and values

These are three important concepts as far as relating theory to practice is concerned. I shall consider each of them in turn before addressing the question of how, in combination, they affect the relationship between theory and practice.

Power

Hugman (1991: 1) argues that:

> Social power is an integral aspect of the daily working lives of

> professionals. The centrality of power in professional work has been increasingly recognised (Wilding, 1982; Cousins, 1987), yet the interconnection of power and caring work in health and welfare provision has been relatively unexplored.

This can also be seen to apply to theory–practice issues, as the concept of power has received relatively little attention in debating such matters. However, power is relevant in a number of ways:

- The 'production of knowledge' is both influenced by, and influential upon, power interests (for example, in terms of who pays for research and who benefits from it).
- Theoretical developments reflect the structure of society in terms of class, race and gender and other such social divisions. That is, theory is predominantly generated by dominant groups in society.
- Human services practice involves the exercise of power. Consequently, the theory base which informs and guides such practice will also have power implications.

These examples reflect just some of the linkages between power and what Sibeon (1991) calls the 'theory-practice problematic'. A further aspect is that of the power of ideas – that is, ideology.

Ideology

The concept of ideology challenges and undermines the simplistic notion that an objective understanding of the world is possible. Ideology shows that some degree of subjective interpretation is inevitable. Donald and Hall (1986: ix–x) argue that:

> . . . the term ideology is used to indicate the frameworks of thought which are used to explain, figure out, make sense of or give meaning to the social and political world. Such ideas do not occur, in social thought, one by one, in an isolated form. They contract links between one another. They define a definite discursive space of meaning which provides us with perspectives on the world, with the particular orientation or frameworks within which we do our thinking. These frameworks both enable us to make sense of perplexing events and relationships – and, inevitably, impose certain 'ways of looking', particular angles of vision, on those events and relationships which we are struggling to make sense of. Without these frameworks, we could not make sense of the world at all. But with them, our perceptions are inevitably structured in a particular direction by the very concepts we are using.

What this passage indicates is that a totally objective theory is not possible. The 'objective' world has to be interpreted through the subjective filter of the framework of ideas by which we make sense of the world (a reflection of the 'dialectical' approach to be discussed in Chapter 4). That is, theories are inevitably influenced by ideologies. This has important implications for the integration of theory and practice, and so it is a point to which I shall return below.

Values

Our interactions with one another and with the world are not neutral or value-free. Our values are those things that are important to us, those that we hold dear. Responding to people's health, welfare and related needs not surprisingly involves values – the fact that we *value* health and social well-being is, in itself, a fundamental issue for understanding the role of values.

There is an expectation that social workers will demonstrate a commitment to certain values in their work:

> – the value and dignity of individuals;
> – the right to respect, privacy and confidentiality;
> – the right of individuals and families to choose;
> – the strengths and skills embodied in local communities;
> – the right to protection of those at risk of abuse and exploitation and violence to themselves and others.
>
> (CCETSW 1991: 16)

This raises two significant issues:

1. Although the above passage relates specifically to social workers, the points covered are more broadly applicable to the human services.
2. There is a clear linkage between the notion of values and that of 'rights'. Indeed, rights are very much part of the value base of human services.

The relationship between theory and practice therefore needs to be seen in the context of values. This will be a key issue in the discussion of philosophy in Chapter 4. Indeed, these three concepts – power, ideology and values – are significant aspects of the context in which both theory and practice operate. What they have in common, of course, is that they are *political* factors. Human services have their roots in politics in a number of ways, and so it would be naïve to assume that the integration of theory and practice is in some way apolitical, although many theorists and researchers have attempted to operate in this way.

In social work, the political context is widely recognized as a significant issue, due in no small part to the influence of radical social work (Corrigan and Leonard 1978; Brake and Bailey 1980), but in nursing and related disciplines, the political dimension is one which has received relatively little attention in the theoretical or practice literature. Dunn (1985: vii) reflects this view when she argues that:

> Many nurses are uncomfortable with the word 'politics'. It belongs to a world of which they do not feel, nor want to be, part. Politics is for others. Politics is a deviant activity in which no self-respecting professional should indulge. Politics, moreover, would wither away if only everything could be discussed and decided on a civilised basis.

The 'head in the sand' approach Dunn describes is one which stands in the way of developing an adequate understanding of theory–practice issues. I shall therefore address it more fully in Chapter 5.

The significance of values in influencing both theory and practice (and indeed the relationship between the two) is a point worth emphasizing. Griseri (1998) argues that values are deeply held and are resistant to change because they *matter.* That is, they are important enough for us to maintain them even in the face of pressure to change them:

> . . . part of being a whole, integrated person is that my values are deeply linked in with many other aspects of my personality. A change in ethics does not, cannot, happen on its own, but must inevitably affect many other elements. Hence the sheer inertia of these means that we hold tenaciously to our values. If one were not so tenacious, one might question how far their ethical views were genuinely held at all.
>
> (1998: 115–16)

We should therefore be careful not to underestimate the important part played by values.

The value of research

Research is an important process through which formal knowledge is developed. It is helpful in two ways, positive and negative. In a positive sense, new knowledge is generated by research activity – both theoretical and empirical – and our practice can often benefit from the new insights and understanding gained, either directly or indirectly. In the negative sense, research can also help us move forward by revealing fallacies and false assumptions. Many things are taken for granted and assumed to be true but do not stand up to rigorous scrutiny when the spotlight of a research study is trained upon them.

Research therefore has a valuable role to play in helping to promote an *informed* approach to human services practice. It provides a basis for reflective practice and a dynamic approach based on continuous learning and development, rather than a static approach based on received wisdom.

However, there are two other points which need to be made in relation to the role and value of research:

1. Different professional groups have different attitudes towards research. In nursing, research tends to be highly valued and its role is accepted with little or no reservation, at a rhetorical level at least. However, in social work the situation is not so clear-cut, as Everitt *et al.* (1992: 1) point out:

   > The relationship between research and social work is problematic. Government committee reports . . . writers . . . and working parties established to address the issue have . . . acknowledged this. Attention has been drawn to social workers not pursuing research, not implementing the findings of research in their practice, nor even reading research reports.

2. Research is not infallible and needs to be treated critically, with a healthy degree of scepticism. An uncritical acceptance of research findings can act as a barrier to the continued development of knowledge as it deters further analysis and learning.

Both of these points are very significant and can be explained by reference to the nature and construction of research, as we shall see in Chapter 3. Both sets of issues relate to more fundamental aspects of research, and need to be seen in a wider context. The important point to note at this stage is that the role of research is a complex and multidimensional one.

Conclusion

This chapter has provided an overview of a number of key issues that have a bearing on the interface of theory and practice. In this way, it has set the scene for the more detailed discussions which appear in the subsequent chapters.

The chapter began with an exposition of Kolb's theory of learning, with its emphasis on learning from experience. One of the major points to emerge from this is that each of us is responsible for our own learning – it is an active process over which we have considerable control. Relating theory to practice can be seen to parallel this process.

From this, I went on to consider the role of professionalism, as the notion of a clear theory base is seen as an integral part of attaining professional status. The concept of professionalism is therefore an important one as far as relating theory to practice is concerned. This is particularly the case in view of the impetus of professional bodies, such as the UKCC and CCETSW, to develop (the use of) the theoretical basis of their respective disciplines.

This led on to a discussion of anti-discriminatory practice and the need for both theory and practice to be underpinned by an understanding of discrimination and oppression and the ways in which these have an impact on the practice of human services workers. This applies in three main ways:

1. Discrimination and oppression play a part – often a major part – in the social, health care or other problems that clients/patients encounter.
2. Intervention can, in itself, result in discrimination and oppression or, at least, condone existing forms and levels of disadvantage.
3. Discrimination and oppression can be inherent in some aspects of policy and theory, as well as practice.

Relating theory to practice therefore needs to take account of the potential for discrimination and oppression and the steps to be taken to develop anti-discriminatory practice.

In order to develop such an approach, both theory and practice have to be seen in a *political* context, particularly with regard to the role of power, ideology and values. Theory is not value-neutral and has to be located within a political framework if we are to avoid a distorted and oversimplified understanding.

Related to this is the need to see research in a broader context. As a source of new knowledge relating directly and indirectly to practice, research has a valuable role to play and has much to offer. However, research raises a number of complex issues and so we should be wary of the not uncommon trap of conceptualizing the role of research in simplistic terms, seeing it as a source of 'hard facts'. What is needed is a more critical approach which recognizes not only the value of research but also its limitations.

This chapter has therefore raised more questions than it answers – a common characteristic of theoretical investigation, but one which prepares the ground for the chapters that follow. In particular, it sets the scene for a fuller understanding of the nature and implications of theory. Indeed, this is the subject matter of Chapter 2.

Food for thought

- Consider your own practice.
  What knowledge do you rely on to carry out your day-to-day work?
  - The law?
  - Social policy?

- Psychological insights about the individual, groups and families?
- Sociological understanding about social institutions and social processes?

◆ Consider your own learning.
What opportunities do you have for learning from your experience?
- Discussion with colleagues?
- Supervision and/or appraisal?
- Training or staff development opportunities?
- Quiet moments for reflection?

◆ Consider your values.
What are the important principles or values that influence your work?
- Religious or spiritual values?
- Political values?
- Moral or ethical principles?
- Your own personal commitment?

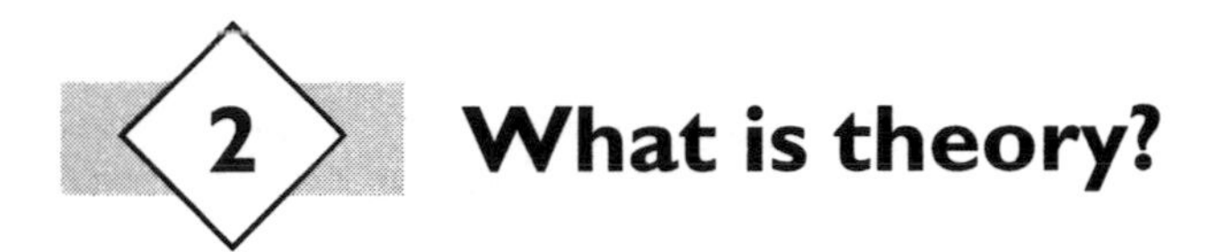

2 What is theory?

Chapter overview

- What is the role of theory?
- What types and levels of theory exist?
- Why is theory important?
- How does theory relate to power?
- What is the 'mystique' of theory?

Introduction

In response to this question of 'What is theory?', Chinn and Kramer (1991: 20) comment:

> Defining 'theory' can be complex, and ultimately most people accept an arbitrary meaning. Just when a definition seems firm, another idea surfaces that must be integrated into it. Like most terms, both within and outside the profession of nursing, theory has common, everyday connotations apparent in such phrases as . . . 'I have a *theory* about that' or . . . 'my *theory* is . . .'. These usages imply that theory is an idea or feeling or that it explains something.

What this passage confirms is that 'theory' is a term used in a variety of ways with no fixed or definitive meaning. However, it would be unwise and unhelpful to leave it at this level of generalization as it is too imprecise for present purposes. What is needed, therefore, is a balance or compromise. The everyday usage of the term is too broad and unfocused, while a narrow and precise definition would be too restrictive and would not reflect the complex and multifaceted nature of the concept.

This chapter attempts to move towards achieving that balance by exploring some of the key aspects of theory as applied to the human services. This will not produce a neat definition, but will provide a much clearer picture of what the term entails and how it can help us understand the complex processes that underpin practice.

Frameworks of understanding

At its simplest level, a theory is an attempt to explain. It is, in short, a framework for understanding. It is a set of ideas linked together to help us make sense of a particular issue or set of issues. It is this notion of a 'network' of ideas that gives us the terms 'theoretical framework' or 'conceptual framework'. It is this combination of ideas to form a framework that acts as the basis of theory. Howe (1987: 10) comments that:

> Theories are not absolute notions of the way things really are, but, so long as they account for what appears to be happening in a way that satisfies the observer, they are retained. They make it intelligible. In a very real way, theory-building is reality-building (Argyris and Schön, 1974, p. 18). Our theories define what we see.

A key word with regard to theory is that of *explanation*, as this is what distinguishes a theory from a model. A model is an intermediate step in the process of theory building. A model seeks to *describe*, for example, by mapping a set of interrelationships. This may show *how* certain factors interrelate, but it will not show *why* they do so – that is where theory comes in. Consider the following example, which shows a model as the intermediate step between determining what needs to be explained and beginning to explain it:

Stage 1: The problematic

This refers to the topic or subject matter chosen as the basis of theoretical enquiry. How and why a certain topic is chosen is, in itself, a major topic in need of explanation, but space does not permit further analysis here. For present purposes, I shall use the example of the sexual division of labour – the ways in which work tasks, both paid and unpaid, are distributed in society according to gender.

Stage 2: The model

The problematic of the sexual division of labour is what needs to be explained. In order to develop our understanding, we need to build up a picture of the component parts of the topic at hand, to get an idea of how the pieces of the jigsaw fit together. In the case of the division of labour, these 'pieces' would include:

- Women do most of the childcare and most of the labour in the home.
- Women are more likely than men to be involved in part-time work.
- Women are more likely to have interrupted work histories (due to childbearing).
- Women have fewer promotion prospects, worse working conditions, less job satisfaction and lower rates of pay.

These jigsaw pieces derive from a range of statistical sources (Equal Opportunities Commission 1987, 1988), but it is only when we start to construct a model that we start to understand their significance and see the interrelationships. That is, by constructing a model we gain additional understanding by virtue of the whole being greater than the sum of its parts.

A model is often expressed in words but can, in many cases, also be shown in diagrammatic form. For example, Figure 2.1 presents the above jigsaw pieces in a diagram which, overall, tells us much more about the sexual division of labour than the individual pieces could. By constructing a model in this way, we gain a much clearer picture of the issues and thereby deepen our understanding.

Stage 3: Theories

Although a model like this is very helpful in showing *how* the sexual division of labour operates, it does not actually tell us *why* it should be so. That is, a model describes but it does not explain. And this is where theories have a part to play, for, as we have noted above, a theory is an attempt to explain, a framework for understanding.

One theoretical explanation for the sexual division of labour would be that of *patriarchy*. Patriarchy refers, literally, to the 'law of the father' and is used as an explanation for male dominance in society. The theory of patriarchy would account for the sexual division of labour by seeing it as part of a broader network of male power and control – a reflection of the way in which power and life-chances are distributed in society according to one's gender.

This is not the only explanation and, indeed, it is rarely, if ever, the case that there is only one explanation for a phenomenon or a set of phenomena. This introduces an important aspect of theory, and one to which I shall return below, namely that theories are *competing* explanations. There will not be a single, definitive theoretical explanation and so, if theory is to be fully understood, a critical and questioning approach will be necessary.

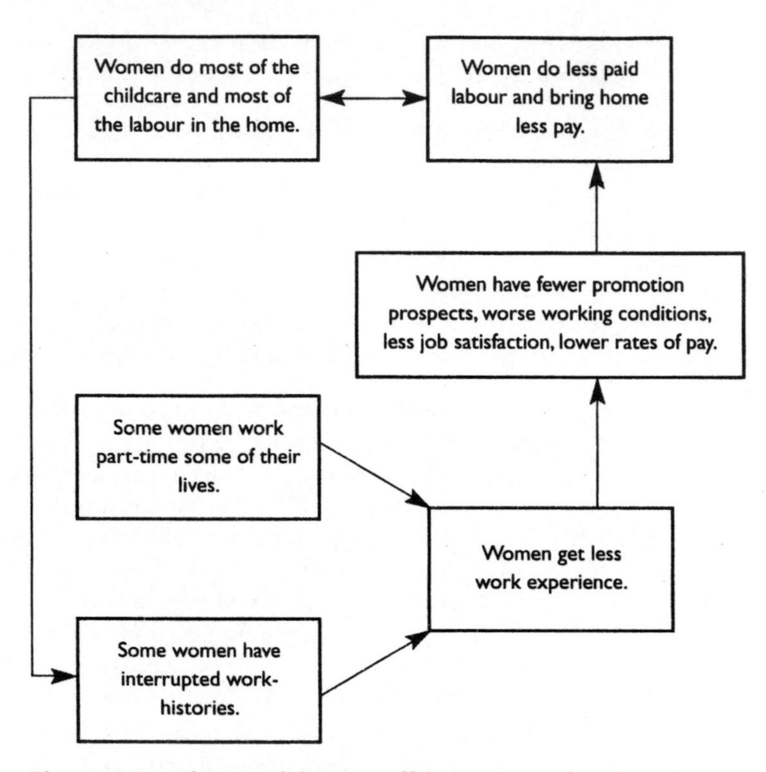

Figure 2.1 The sexual division of labour. Reproduced, with permission, from Chamberlain *et al.* (1990)

This conception of a theory as a framework is captured in the following passage from Compton and Galaway (1979: 41, quoted in Roberts 1990: 17):

> A theory is a coherent group of general propositions or concepts used as principles of explanation for a class of phenomena – a more or less verified or established explanation accounting for known facts or phenomena and their inter-relationship. If one thinks of knowledge as discrete bits of truth or discrete facts and observations like a pile of bricks, theory can be likened to a wall of bricks. In a theory the observations of the real world are ordered and put together in a certain way and held together by certain assumptions or hypotheses as bricks in a wall are held together by a material that cements them in place. Thus theory is a coherent group of general propositions, containing both confirmed and assumptive knowledge, held together by connective notions that seek to explain in a rational way the observed facts of phenomena and the relationship of these phenomena to each other.

However, Roberts points out that this definition takes no account of the values of the theorist. It gives the impression that theorizing is an objective process independent of the value position of the theorist. In this sense, Compton and Galaway's conception of theory goes a step beyond the basic notion of a framework for understanding and implies that such understanding can be objective and value-free. That is, they are implicitly adopting a *scientific* conception of theory. This is an important issue which will reappear later in this chapter and will be addressed more fully in Chapter 3.

Types and levels of theory

To develop a comprehensive typology of theories would be a major undertaking and is far beyond the scope of this book. However, we can usefully explore some of the major types and levels of theory in order to take our understanding of these issues forward.

A good way to begin this is to explain the distinction between grand theories and middle-range theories. A grand theory is one that attempts to explain more or less everything in society. That is, it goes beyond a simple level of explanation and becomes a philosophy of life, a particular view of the world, or to use the technical term, a *Weltanschauung*. Examples of grand theories would be psychodynamics, marxism and existentialism.

Middle-range theories are less ambitious in their claims and attempt to explain only a limited range of phenomena. That is, their focus is much narrower and their scope is not so all-embracing. Symbolic interactionism is a good example of a middle-range theory. It seeks to explain interpersonal interactions but remains silent on the questions of wider social issues. This raises two significant points:

1. Middle-range theories are often unfairly criticized for being limited in the scope of their analysis. Such criticism is unfair in so far as it involves criticizing the theorists for not covering something they were not trying to cover!
2. Middle-range theories are 'safer' than grand theories in two senses. First, they make fewer claims and are therefore less likely to be proven wrong. Second, by definition they have little or nothing to say about wider social factors such as power, inequality, oppression and disadvantage. They are therefore less likely to be seen as a threat to the powers that be and the status quo.

In addition to grand and middle-range theories, there are also micro-theories. These are on a very small scale and seek to explain only a very limited range of phenomena. Berger and Kellner (1981) are subtly critical of the tendency, in sociology at least, for such small-scale studies to proliferate at the expense of what they call the 'big questions':

> Good sociologists have always had an insatiable curiosity about even the trivialities of human behaviour, and if this curiosity leads a sociologist to devote many years to the painstaking exploration of some small corner of the social world that may appear quite trivial to others, so be it: Why do more teenagers pick their noses in rural Minnesota than in rural Iowa? . . . Far be it from us to denigrate such research interests!
>
> (Berger and Kellner 1981: 15–16)

Grand theories have been criticized by a number of thinkers who subscribe to what can broadly be defined as a postmodern approach (see, for example, Hollinger 1994). However, Sibeon (1996: 3) counters this view:

> . . . there is a danger of an overreaction against grand generalizations. Nomothetic (or generalizing) forms of knowledge refer to categories of persons, places, events etc.; ideographic (or particularizing) knowledge refers to a particular person, place or event. The social sciences deal mainly in nomothetic knowledge; this is acceptable, indeed necessary . . . [S]ocial science generalizations are entirely appropriate, provided they are of more limited scope than the generalizations associated with grand theory.

This distinction between *nomothetic* and *ideographic* theories is also an important distinction to consider in its own right. As the above passage suggests, a nomothetic approach is one which seeks to generalize, to identify broad patterns, principles and recurring themes. An ideographic approach, by contrast, is one which focuses more narrowly on a particular set of phenomena and does not seek to generalize far beyond those particular circumstances. In this regard, nomothetic theory is concerned mainly with *breadth* – that is, with developing a broader theoretical understanding based on principles and patterns that should also apply in other circumstances – while an ideographic approach focuses on *depth* – seeking a fairly in-depth understanding of a particular issue or topic but without wishing to extend that understanding more broadly.

A similarly helpful and related distinction between types of theory that can be drawn is that between sensitizing theory and substantive theory. Sibeon (1996: 4) again makes apt comment when he argues that:

> Substantive theories aim to provide us with new empirical information, whereas sensitizing theoretical frameworks are

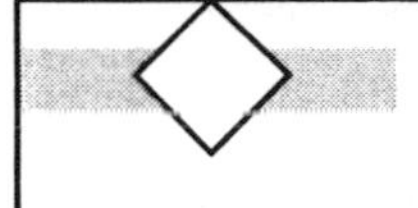

Practice Focus 2.1

When Sarah joined the multidisciplinary team working with people with a learning disability, she soon became disillusioned. She very quickly learned that the team operated exclusively within a behaviourist framework. Although she was comfortable with this type of approach, she was also used to drawing on a much broader range of tools of intervention, as her hospital-based training introduced students to a number of different approaches without specializing in any one in particular. She felt guilty that she had not 'done her homework' to find out how the team operated before accepting the post.

> intended to furnish general orientations or perspectives; they are intended to equip us with ways of thinking about the world.

In Chapter 4 we shall explore the significance of philosophy in general and existentialism in particular, and this distinction can also be seen to apply to the discussions there.

Another important issue to consider in looking at types of theory is the concept of a *paradigm*. A paradigm is a theoretical approach which encompasses a number of related theories: 'Theories can be grouped together within various perspectives. These perspectives are known as "paradigms". For example, behaviourism is a paradigm which subsumes the various forms of behavioural theory' (Thompson 1992a: 13).

Parse (1987) illustrates the notion of paradigm by distinguishing between what she calls the 'Man-environment totality paradigm' and the 'Man-environment simultaneity paradigm'. The former refers to a view of the person ('man') as a 'mechanistic organism who adapts to the environment and strives towards a state of well-being', whereas the latter refers to a different view of the person, namely a 'unitary being in continuous mutual interrelationship with the environment, and whose health is a negentropic unfolding' (1987: 4). The actual difference between these two issues is not the most important question for present purposes. What *is* important is to note that different paradigms are based on different sets of assumptions and therefore have different implications and outcomes. As Parse (1987: 2) comments:

> Theories are grounded in the belief system of the paradigm, which means that the definition of the concepts of the theories are congruent with beliefs set forth in the paradigm. Theories of a paradigm are the specific tools that guide practice and research.

	'FORMAL' THEORY	'INFORMAL' THEORY
1. THEORIES OF WHAT SOCIAL WORK IS.	Formal written paradigms which define the nature and purposes of welfare e.g. personal pathology, liberal reform, marxist, feminist, etc.	Moral–political cultural values of welfare internalised by practitioners and drawn upon for defining the nature and purposes ('functions') of social work in society.
2. THEORIES OF HOW TO DO SOCIAL WORK.	Formal written *theories of practice*, e.g. casework methods theory, family therapy or groupwork or community work theories of practice.	Inductively derived and usually unwritten informal *practice theories* constructed experientially from the practical experience of 'doing' social work.
3. THEORIES OF THE CLIENT WORLD.	Formal written social science theories and empirical data on personality, social behaviour, marriage, the family, class, gender, race, community, deviancy, etc.	Practitioners' use of experientially acquired general culture meanings and definitions of (for example) the nature of social behaviour, class, race, 'the family' as an institution, 'normal' behaviour, cultural definitions of 'good' or 'bad' parenting, and cultural assumptions about (say) the 'proper' roles of women in society.

Figure 2.2 Sibeon's typology of theories. Reproduced, with permission, from Sibeon (1990)

Once again, we see that theoretical enterprises are not objective and value-free but are clearly grounded in sets of beliefs, values and assumptions.

Another aspect of understanding types and levels of theory is discussed by Sibeon (1990). Building on the work of Timms and Timms (1977), he outlines a three-level classification of (social work) theory, based on theories of:

- what social work is;
- how to do social work;
- the nature of the client world.

When this threefold classification is further subdivided in terms of formal and informal theory (a distinction I shall discuss in more detail below), a six-cell matrix is produced, as shown in Figure 2.2. This can be a helpful framework for understanding some of the complexities of theory by showing in a clear and simple form some of the ways in

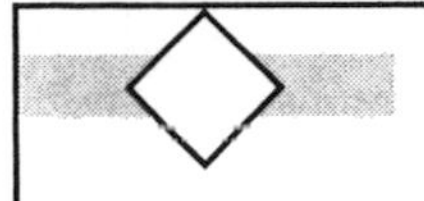

Practice Focus 2.2

When her employers introduced an appraisal scheme, Tina was asked to review her previous learning and begin to identify her training needs. When she began to do this, she was quite amazed to realize how much she had learned by being part of an experienced staff group and working alongside skilled and knowledgeable colleagues.

However, at her first appraisal interview, discussion centred on how she could maximize her learning and her effectiveness. It was only at this point that she realized that, although she had 'absorbed' a great deal of learning by working alongside experienced colleagues, she could in fact have learned a great deal more if she had adopted a more proactive approach to learning and had used her colleagues as a resource, rather than simply as implicit role models.

which elements of theory interrelate. It can also be generalized beyond social work to be made more applicable to nursing and the other human services if appropriate modifications are made.

The distinction between formal and informal theory is also a helpful one, as it takes us another step forwards towards making sense of the complex world of theory. Curnock and Hardiker (1979) draw a distinction between formal 'theories of practice' and informal 'practice theories'. The former type of theory is 'official' theory in the sense that it is formally recorded in academic literature and forms the basis of much formal teaching. Informal 'practice theories', by contrast, are not officially recognized or formally codified. They constitute the 'practice wisdom' of a profession, the informal knowledge and assumptions which are 'built up through actual practice and "culturally transmitted" to new recruits to the profession' (Thompson 1992a: 12). This idea is captured, in a nursing context, by the notion of 'Sister says'. That is, much of this practice wisdom is learned by working alongside more experienced colleagues.

Both types of theory have advantages and disadvantages relative to each other. In terms of direct applicability to practice, informal theory scores more highly than formal theory in so far as it addresses more specifically and directly day-to-day practice issues. Such theory was born of practice and is therefore closely linked to the everyday concerns and realities of practitioners. Formal theory, by contrast, is at one remove from actual practice but scores highly in terms of being explicit and therefore open to question. It is possible to take issue with formal theory and challenge its basis; it can be adapted and extended by rational analysis, discussion and empirical investigation. However, informal theory, because of its status as received wisdom, is far less open to challenge:

> Whereas formal theory is open to debate, examination and counterargument, informal theory is relatively unassailable insofar as it is covert, implicit and taken for granted as 'obvious' or 'common sense'. In other words, informal theory has the status of dogma. Dogma is not based on evidence, coherent argument or experimental testing, nor is it open to critical analysis as it is taken for granted as 'obvious' or just 'common sense'.
>
> (Thompson 1992a: 18)

Both types of theory have a role to play but both also have limitations. Chapter 5 will examine some of the ways in which these limitations can be addressed and their impact minimized. For example, Coutts-Jarman (1993: 78) comments that:

> Benner (1984) talks of the 'wealth of untapped knowledge embedded in the practices and "know-how" of expert nurse clinicians'. She states that for this knowledge to expand and develop nurses need to record systematically what they learn from their own experience. While nurses continue to describe their actions, clinical skills and decisions as intuition, clinical expertise will continue to go unrecognised and a knowledge base of nursing skills will not develop.

This is an important observation, as it points out the wasted opportunities implicit in the tendency to reject theory and 'stick to practice'. As we shall see in Chapter 5, theory and practice are closely interwoven, and so we need to understand not only how theory influences practice, but also how practice can, and should, influence theory. In sum, we can make better use of theory not only by making formal theory more applicable to practice, but also by making informal theory more open to scrutiny, debate and development.

These, then, are some of the main types and levels of theory, although we have by no means covered them all. By now it should be clear that theory is a broad term which covers a wide range of elements and component parts. It is beyond the scope of this book to present a comprehensive analysis of theory but, none the less, there are other important aspects we can explore, beginning with: 'Why is theory important?'

The importance of theory

Theory is important for the human services in a number of ways. I shall outline some of these here so that we can more firmly establish the significance of theory for practice.

Anti-discriminatory practice

In Chapter 1, a case was made for using theory to contribute to the development of anti-discriminatory practice. Indeed, theory has a very important role to play in this respect in terms of its capacity for 'debunking'. This is a term used in sociology to refer to a process of 'unmasking' social reality by looking at the complex social processes that go on beneath the surface of social life. It is part of what Mills (1970) calls the 'sociological imagination', the ability to see beyond the narrow confines of everyday thought. This involves understanding individuals as part of wider social and political patterns and structures. As Mills (1970: 32) comments, the sociological imagination is a: 'quality of mind that seems most dramatically to promise an understanding of the intimate realities of ourselves in connexion with larger social realities'. Theory helps us to 'debunk' narrow, commonsensical explanations of social behaviour and allows it to be seen in the broader context of social processes and structures. In this sense, theory is a counterbalance to the tendency to rely uncritically on a commonsense conception of people and their problems. That is, the use of theory implies a critique of common sense.

This critique can be seen to be based on the inadequacy of 'common sense' as an explanatory framework for human services practice. This inadequacy is based on four key factors:

> First, it is contradictory. Common sense proverbs are an example of this. Compare 'Out of sight, out of mind' with 'Absence makes the heart grow fonder'. Psychology can explain this contradiction by pointing out that research shows that the former applies to extraverts whereas the latter applies to introverts (cf. Eysenck, 1965). This explanation derives from psychological theory and not from common sense itself. The use of common sense is therefore limited.
>
> Second, common sense is ideological – it serves to reinforce traditional values and the inequalities associated with these. It is based on implicit assumptions and if we rely on such common sense to guide our thoughts we are not in a position to question those assumptions (Thompson, 1990a). Common sense therefore deters critical thinking. Third, common sense is 'culture-bound'. That is, what is taken for granted in one culture may not be considered the same way within a different cultural setting. This is particularly important in our multiracial context.
>
> Fourth, common sense does not always provide answers to the questions we need to ask ... For example, when dealing with a child at risk, common sense is not a sufficient guide in deciding whether the child should remain at home. If it were simply a

> matter of 'common sense' training and experience in child protection would not be needed.
>
> (Thompson 1992a: 12)

This passage illustrates the range of dangers inherent in relying on common sense but it is the second point in particular which has a bearing on anti-discriminatory practice. Common sense is imbued with discriminatory and oppressive assumptions – that women belong at home, that black people are inferior and so on. A practice which relies on common sense is one which runs a very strong risk of legitimating and reinforcing discrimination and oppression. As Sayer (1992) explains, common sense has a tendency to 'naturalize' social phenomena, to make them seem normal and natural and therefore beyond question.

Theories, too, can be discriminatory and oppressive, but an approach based explicitly and openly on a theoretical perspective at least has the *potential* to counter oppression and develop anti-discriminatory practice, whereas common sense offers only barriers to doing so.

The fallacy of theoryless practice

Timms (1968: 23) makes the point that: 'We cannot conceive of practice without employing some kind of theory about what constitutes the practice, what indicates good or bad practice and so on'. Pilalis (1986: 92) adds weight to this argument by commenting that: '"Practice" cannot be devoid of theory. Similarly, it is difficult to conceive of "theory" which is "purely" descriptive and devoid of a reference to purposeful action'. The same point – that theory and practice are inextricably linked – is also made by Curnock and Hardiker (1979), Sibeon (1990) and a number of other writers.

When practitioners comment that they 'prefer to stick to practice', as if practice can be divorced from theory, they are reflecting the 'fallacy of theoryless practice' (Thompson 1992a). They are assuming, quite inappropriately, that complex actions can be divorced from thought. Underpinning their fallacy is the notion that theory refers only to formal 'book theory', that informal theory either does not exist or does not count. As we noted earlier, informal, 'uncodified' theory has an important part to play in guiding our actions and informing our practice.

If we do not recognize that frameworks of ideas and values are influencing how we act and interact, we are not in a position to question those ideas and ensure that they are appropriate and constructive. That is, we need to recognize the fallacy of theoryless practice so that we are not guilty of failing to review our ideas and lacking the flexibility to adapt or abandon them in the light of changing circumstances. In short, we need to be wary of the fallacy of theoryless practice, as it leads to dogmatism and stands in the way of the development of reflective practice. As Howe (1987: 9) comments:

> To travel at all is to hold ideas about the behavioural and social terrain over which we journey. To show no interest in . . . theory is simply to travel blind. This is bad for practice and unhelpful to clients.

Failing to recognize the role of underpinning theory and values can lead to 'dangerous practice' (Thompson and Bates 1998) in the sense that misguided interventions may not only fail to be effective but may also make the situation worse:

> The fact that many workers do not explicitly apply theory to practice does not mean that they are not relying on a theory base. What it does mean is that they are drawing on ideas in an implicit, indirect and unsystematic way. At worst, therefore, 'I prefer to stick to practice' can mean 'I prefer to act without thinking' or 'I prefer not to question the basis of my practice'.
>
> Clearly, this is not an attitude conducive to professional development, nor does it provide any safeguards against bad practice. Needless to say, this attitude is therefore a very dangerous one.
>
> (Thompson and Bates 1995: 57)

Evaluation

Human services work is undertaken with particular goals in mind. That is, they comprise purposive activities. This raises the question of evaluation – studying, and where possible, measuring the effectiveness of interventions and the factors that have contributed to, or stood in the way of, such effectiveness. This process is extremely difficult, if not impossible, to implement without a theory base from which to operate.

Evaluation can be seen to be theory-dependent in a number of ways:

1. The process itself reflects a theoretical orientation akin to principles of strategic management (the importance of setting objectives and measuring progress towards them; see Asch and Bowman 1989).
2. The identification of problems and the subsequent setting of objectives will, in itself, reflect a theoretical orientation. For example, how a worker responds to a person experiencing depression will depend, to a large extent, on the theoretical perspective adopted (ranging from depression as an illness to depression as a response to oppression).
3. The methods of intervention chosen will also reflect the worker's

theoretical understanding of the situation and how best to respond to it (counselling, drug therapy, environmental change and so on).
4. The implementation of such methods is also theory-dependent in so far as the worker's understanding of his or her role *vis-à-vis* the service user can have major implications in terms of the outcome of interventions. For example, in child protection work, a practitioner who sees the parents as 'inadequate' is likely to receive a different response compared with a colleague who adopts a broader, less pathologizing perspective.

Theory is therefore important as an underpinning part of the process of evaluation. A practice which is open to evaluation – and the lessons that can be learned from this – is a practice which owes much to theory.

Continuous professional development

An important source of motivation for human services workers is that of continuous professional development. This involves adopting an attitude of continually learning from our experience and thereby avoiding becoming complacent or 'getting into a rut'. Part of this process is to avoid unthinking routines which produce unthinking routine practice of a superficial nature, and to develop a more critical approach informed by reflection (Thompson and Bates 1998). Powell (1989b: 38) comments on this in relation to nursing: 'Certainly nurses are beginning to recognise the satisfaction to be gained from a more in-depth approach to patient problems, and we are rejecting routinised practices to a greater extent than a few years ago'.

Theory is an important ingredient in maintaining continuous professional development – constantly seeking opportunities for learning and development. This helps to avoid what Schön (1983) refers to as 'overlearning', as Powell (1989a: 825) explains:

> As practice becomes routine, the practitioner may fail to think about his [*sic*] work and fall into rigid repetition. He may also fail to be aware of phenomena which do not fit his categories of theories-in-use. Schön refers to this as 'selective inattention' and describes both rigidity and lack of awareness as overlearning . . .

Theories provide frameworks of explanation so that we can make sense of new experiences and develop our understanding of the world, rather than distort such experiences by forcing them into existing, but perhaps inadequate, patterns of understanding.

This notion of continuous professional development is an important one, and one to which we shall return in Chapter 5 in relation to the importance of 'reflection-in-action' as a strategy for relating theory to practice.

Professional accountability

The provision of human services involves considerable public expenditure, as well as charitable and other contributions. Also, and more importantly, such provision has major implications in terms of people's quality of life and, indeed, often in terms of life and death. Consequently, there are built-in safeguards of accountability which require staff to be able to justify their actions. Such actions include appraisal systems, statutory reviews, complaints procedures and formal inquiries.

When called upon to account for our actions, it is, of course, important that we are able to provide a *rationale* to justify our actions. Responses of the 'it seemed a good idea at the time' kind are unlikely to hold any water. What is required is an account of practice grounded in an explanatory framework which:

- clarifies the basis of the intervention and the objectives set;
- explains the actions taken to meet the objectives and the reasons for doing so;
- evaluates the intervention.

In short, the account needs to be based on theory. This is confirmed by the Department of Health (1988: 12) guide to child protection assessment, which regards acting 'without a theoretical base and systematic, structured approach to intervention' as an aspect of professional dangerousness, a barrier to effective practice.

Inappropriate responses

A failure to draw on theoretical knowledge may lead to an inappropriate response on the part of the worker. We may misinterpret what is happening and react in a way which is not helpful or which even makes the situation worse. For example, a person experiencing a bereavement may express considerable anger towards the worker. If the worker does not recognize such anger as a common part of the grieving process, he or she could easily misread the situation and interpret the anger as a rejection of the worker's help (Lendrum and Syme 1992).

Similarly, we may simply not know how to respond in certain circumstances. While an explicitly theory-based approach by no means guarantees an appropriate response, it does give a framework for analysing the situation and generating a number of possible options. Indeed, it is not uncommon for explicit theory to be used in this way, as a fall-back position in times of difficulty, that is when workers feel 'stuck' – 'useful "reserves" to back up the routine use of implicit knowledge' (Thompson 1991a: 29).

Clearly, then, there are many important reasons why theory has a significant role to play, why it is important in terms of maximizing the effectiveness of practice. A discussion of the ways in which the use of theory can be enhanced is a central part of Chapter 5 and so we shall revisit some of these issues there.

The bias of theory

In Chapter 1, the point was made that theories are inevitably influenced by ideologies and linked to power relations in wider society. Theorizing is by no means a 'pure' activity, detached from the reality of the social and political world. That is, theory is inevitably embedded in the social context in which it arises and in which it should be used. As Sayer (1992) argues, any attempt to explain social phenomena necessarily involves a process of evaluating them. Society and social science theory are necessarily intertwined, a point I shall develop more fully in Chapter 3.

The social context of theory is reflected in the biases apparent in traditional theory. For example, consider the feminist concept of '*her*story', the critique of the invisibility of women in (men's) accounts of history. As Miles (1989: 11) comments:

> 'What is history?' brooded Gibbon, the great historian of the Roman Empire. Little more than a register of the crimes, follies and misfortunes of men? At that the hand that rocks the cradle has taken up the pen to set the record straight. In history, there were women too.

The relative absence of women in accounts of history reflects male dominance in society in terms of both the power struggles described in history texts and the authorship of those texts as primarily a male activity. History is therefore not neutral, but rather reflects the patriarchal structure of society.

Patriarchy is a very significant term in this context, as the 'law of the father' subordinates not only women but also children. Stainton Rogers and Stainton Rogers (1992) therefore argue that children, too, are largely 'invisible' in the accounts of history dominated by patriarchal ideology.

Pascall (1986) also challenges patriarchy when she applies a similar argument to social policy, indicating that women's voices are rarely heard, despite the fact that women make up the majority of welfare consumers and providers. She goes on to argue that the ideology underpinning the Welfare State has contributed to the subordination of women:

> The Welfare State, then, may be seen as public control of the private sphere, and increasing male control of female work.

> Most obviously, the biology of reproduction has become the property of male medicine. But the family has also lost control of significant aspects of reproductive work to the male-dominated professions of medicine, teaching and social work. And by supporting the breadwinner/dependant form of family, with the woman at home, social policy has played a part in controlling women, keeping them in the private sphere and out of public life.
>
> (Pascall 1986: 25)

Williams (1989) echoes this view and reinforces the critique of traditional social policy as a male preserve. She also extends the argument to include a racial dimension by emphasizing the ethnocentric nature of dominant thinking in social policy. She comments on the tendency to neglect issues of ethnicity and racism as well as gender:

> In general 'race' and gender are issues that have been neglected or marginalised in the discipline of social policy, particularly in terms of a failure to, first, acknowledge the experiences and struggles of women and of Black people over welfare provision; secondly, to account for racism and sexism in the provision of state welfare; thirdly, to give recognition to work which *does* attempt to analyse the relationship between the welfare state and the oppressions of women and of Black people (and, historically, other racialized groups like the Irish and the Jews); and fourthly, to work out a progressive welfare strategy which incorporates the needs and demands which emerge from such strategies and analyses.
>
> (Williams 1989: xi)

What both Pascall and Williams are promoting is a critique of the biases inherent in traditional social policy analysis. This can also be extended to take account of issues of disability, age, sexual identity and so on. The central point to be emphasized is that the theory base underpinning social policy reflects the biases and interests of dominant power groups and therefore indicates the operation of ideology (see also Smith 1998).

One aspect of ideology of relevance here is its tendency to define the problematic, to influence what is to be studied and how. In this way, dominant ideologies within the human services have a tendency to marginalize issues of sexism, racism and other forms of discrimination and oppression. This is a very important aspect of ideology and is again a matter of power. As Benton (1981: 163) comments: 'The power to prevent issues and conflict from surfacing may be one of the most insidious forms of political power of all'.

What this tells us, then, in terms of our basic question of 'What is theory?', is that it is *not* an abstract academic exercise unconnected with the real world; it is, rather, a dynamic development of ideas linked to power structures in society and the interaction of dominant and countervailing ideological forces.

Evaluating theories

While no single theory can be expected to provide definitive answers or 'ultimate truths', we should not fall into the trap of going to the other extreme in assuming that any theory is as good as another. There are ways of evaluating the respective contribution of different theories and I shall outline one particular approach to such evaluation here. Drawing on the work of Sibeon (1996; 1999), we can identify four 'cardinal sins' of theorizing – that is, four particular ways in which the value of a theory as an explanatory framework can be undermined.

Reductionism

Reductionism is a form of oversimplification in which a phenomenon which operates at a number of levels is explained solely in terms of only one such level. For example, racism can be seen to operate on at least three levels (personal, cultural and structural), and so to conceptualize it purely in terms of personal prejudice is profoundly reductionist and therefore theoretically invalid (see Thompson 1998a).

Essentialism

This refers to the tendency to regard fluid, changeable phenomena as if they were fixed and rigid ('essences'). This leads to various forms of determinism in which human agency is ignored or marginalized in favour of other forces which are assumed to be the causes of our behaviour (heredity, upbringing, destiny and so on). This is discussed further in Chapter 4.

Reification

To 'reify' means literally to turn into a thing, to treat as an entity in its own right. Reification therefore involves attributing agency or decision-making capabilities to phenomena which have no such ability. For example, what Sibeon (1996) refers to as 'taxonomic collectivities' (women, black people, the working class) are not entities that can make decisions or carry out actions in their own right. That is, while individual women or groups of women can act and make decisions, the overall category of 'women' cannot act in a unified way as if they had just one voice. Terms like 'women', 'ethnic minorities' are generalizations and cannot therefore legitimately be treated as active agents in their own right. Therefore, when a theorist begins a statement with a phrase like, 'Women . . .', we should be asking whether this is intended to refer to some women, most women or all women.

Teleology

A 'teleological' explanation is one which confuses cause and effect by assuming an underlying purpose. For example, some forms of functionalist sociology would describe the family as having the 'function' or 'purpose' of socializing children. While not wishing to dispute that the family has a role in socialization, to conceptualize this in terms of a function or purpose is to confuse something which has developed historically (and is therefore the *effect* of human behaviour over a number of generations) with a predefined role or purpose (a cause). As Sibeon (1999: 318) comments:

> Functional *teleology* refers to illicit attempts to explain the causes of social phenomena in terms of their effects; the point to be made here is that in the absence of intentional planning by actors somewhere, sometime, it is a teleological fallacy to attempt to explain the causes of social phenomena in terms of their effects (Betts 1986: 51).

What we need to do, therefore, in order to be clear about the merits or otherwise of a particular theory is to check whether it is flawed in terms of one or more of these weaknesses. We therefore need to ask whether the explanation given is sufficiently sophisticated or whether it:

- reduces a multilevel phenomenon to a single-level explanation (reductionism);
- mistakes fluid, open processes (such as personal identity) for fixed, unchanging entities (essentialism);
- treats descriptive generalizations as if they were agents capable of making decisions and acting in a purposeful way (reification);
- regards the effects of history (current social practices, for example) as if they were the cause of social phenomena according to a predefined function or purpose (teleology).

The mystique of theory

Understanding the nature and operation of theory is a complex undertaking of major proportions, as is evidenced by the success of this chapter in providing only a very sketchy outline of the parameters of theory. This complexity is part of the foundation of the mystique which has grown up around theory and now acts as a barrier to many practitioners drawing more fruitfully on a more explicit theory base. However, this complexity is not the only foundation of the mystique of theory and so, before leaving the question of 'What is theory?', it is worth highlighting some of the other elements which create this barrier of mystique.

A simple way of understanding the mystique of theory is to divide the blame between theorists and practitioners. On the one hand, many academic writers have contributed to the mystique by presenting theory in a highly abstract, inaccessible form, which can have the effect of alienating practitioners. This is not to bemoan the use of jargon, for in discussing and analysing the social world, technical terms are necessary in order to distinguish social science concepts from everyday, common-sense terms. However, the legitimate use of jargon has often been exceeded to the point of mystification, thus widening the gap between theory and practice. Similarly, some academic enterprises can, arguably, be seen to have more in common with intellectual game-playing than breaking down barriers between theory and practice (for example, Curt 1994).

On the other hand, many practitioners have also contributed to this gap by adopting a position of anti-intellectualism by rejecting the value of theory. This is particularly the case in social work, as Sibeon (1991: 9) suggests:

> ... academic knowledge has been 'incorrectly' taught by academics, nor is it because of any idiosyncratic or personal 'incompetence' on the part of particular social work students and practitioners: it is because the socially constructed reality of social work practice in general is such that formal academic knowledge ... is simply not 'required' for social work practice.

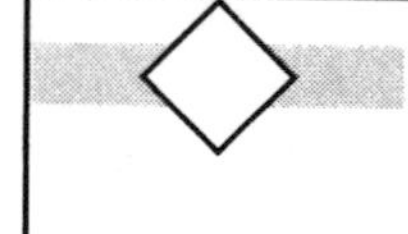

Practice Focus 2.3

Howard had been a very keen student on his social work course and felt he had learned a great deal. Moreover, he was looking forward to having the opportunity to continue his learning and professional development as a qualified worker. However, his first job after qualifying presented him with a major dilemma. In his first supervision session, his team leader advised him to 'Put the last two years behind you – we don't work like that here'.

cont.

Practice Focus 2.3 (*cont.*)

Understandably, Howard felt totally demoralized and undermined by this attitude, and this was reflected in his practice, temporarily at least, as he lacked confidence and became indecisive. Ironically, this only served to reinforce the team leader's mistrust of theory, as he saw Howard's problems as a reflection of his being 'too theoretical' and therefore not adequately equipped for practice.

Fortunately, Howard realized what was happening and was able to move on to another team where he flourished in an atmosphere which encouraged learning and development. He often wondered, though, how many others had not been so fortunate and had become trapped in a demoralizing work environment which sapped their appetite for learning and their creativity.

This resistance to formal theory manifests itself in a number of ways, some overt ('forget that college nonsense, you're in the real world now') and some more subtle, reflecting a set of cultural norms at odds with the ethos of professional education and training.

This notion of culture is an important one, for what this discussion of mystique reveals is, to a certain extent at least, a clash of cultures. Schön (1992) captures the difference between the two cultures in terms of his distinction between the 'high ground' of research-based theory and technique and the 'swampy lowlands' of day-to-day problems and concerns. That is, the two groups – academics and practitioners – have different interests and different starting points, or, to use a technical term, they operate within different discourses (Rojek *et al.* 1988).

There are, of course, historical reasons for the development of the two cultures, reasons which require a more detailed analysis than space permits here. However, it is important to note that the differences in culture are very significant in terms of the mystique of theory. Challenging that mystique, and breaking down some of the cultural barriers, will be part of the discussions which will go to make up Chapters 5 and 7.

Conclusion

As we have seen, there can be no simple or straightforward answer to the question of 'What is theory?' We can, however, take significant steps forward towards narrowing the gap between theory and practice by understanding some of the key elements of theory as the basis for informed, sensitive and critical practice.

A key aspect of this, but one not yet discussed in any detail, is the nature and role of scientific thought. To what extent and in what ways can theory be said to be scientific? What does it mean to say that practice is based on 'scientific knowledge' and what implications does this have? These are some of the important questions that need to be addressed. They therefore feature as a significant part of Chapter 3, where the focus of analysis is on social science as a basis for human services practice. It is to these issues that we now turn.

Food for thought

- Consider the role of theory.
  - What theoretical perspectives have an influence on your practice, directly or indirectly?
  - What are the key points from these theories that inform your thinking on practice issues?
  - How did you learn about these?
  - Have they changed over time?
- Consider the types and levels of theory.
  - Is there a 'grand' or overarching theory that underpins your practice?
  - If so, is this linked to a particular value base?
  - What are your views about the nature and purpose of your particular professional discipline (your 'theory of what it is')?
- Consider the importance of theory.
  - Do you have opportunities to evaluate your work?
  - If not, are you able to create any?
  - How can you ensure that you do not lose sight of the value of theory as a basis for practice?

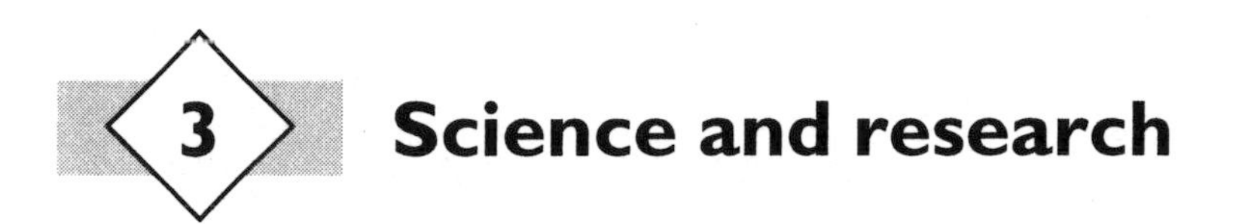

3 Science and research

Chapter overview

- What is science?
- Is science value-free?
- What is the role of research?
- How do we know whether research is valid?
- What is 'research-minded practice'?

Introduction

To describe one's work as 'scientific' is to claim a certain amount of prestige for its status. 'Scientific' knowledge is seen, in general terms, as not just different from other forms of knowledge, but actually superior to them. In this respect, then, the theoretical bases of the human services can be seen to gain in status from having the label 'scientific' applied to them. As Smith (1998: 29) comments: 'the idea of being "scientific" provides additional meaning and a sense of truth, authenticity and the stamp of authority'.

However, as this chapter will demonstrate, the situation is not quite so simple and the notion of scientific status is a problematical one. The relationship between the natural sciences and the human services is one that can be seen to have been overemphasized, while the role of social science has not always been fully appreciated. This is particularly the case in nursing, although the same issues do arise in other forms of human service, albeit in slightly different guises.

This chapter addresses the question of 'positivism', the view that the human or social sciences can follow the same patterns and methodology as the natural sciences, and highlights the major weaknesses in adopting this approach to human services issues and concerns. A more appropriate form of scientific inquiry is outlined and the implications of this are considered. Following on from this, the nature, value and limitations of research are examined and the notion of 'research-minded practice' is endorsed as a useful way forward.

The critique of positivism

Positivism is a term used to describe a particular approach to science, whether natural or social science. It is characterized by a number of key features:

- The belief that universal laws (of nature or of society) can be discovered by scientific investigation.
- A commitment to 'objective', observable and measurable factors and a mistrust, or even total rejection, of subjective factors.
- A view of science as a morally neutral or value-free enterprise.
- A commitment to empirical research as the most appropriate form of scientific investigation.

With specific reference to *social* science, there is an additional aspect to consider, namely the view that social science is a parallel endeavour to that of the natural sciences. Smith (1998: 77) describes positivism in the following terms:

> Positivist approaches to the social sciences claim the label scientific, for they assume things can be studied as hard facts and the relationship between these facts established as scientific laws. For positivists, such laws have the status of truth and social objects can be studied in much the same way as natural objects.

Heather (1976: 13), writing in a similar vein, argues that the distinguishing feature of positivism is 'the attempt to apply to the affairs of man [*sic*] the methods and principles of the natural sciences'.

This is a very significant issue for, as I shall emphasize below, this amounts to a serious distortion of social science as a basis for the human services practice. It tries to squeeze social and psychological phenomena into an inappropriate frame of reference.

Positivism has been a major influence in the philosophy of science over a significant period of time. Although less dominant now than in the past, positivism remains a pervasive influence at both an explicit and implicit level. It is therefore important to be clear about the problems inherent in adopting a positivist approach, so that we are not carried along uncritically by the force of positivist tradition. I shall tackle each of the key aspects in turn, highlighting significant weaknesses.

Universal laws

A central tenet of positivism is the existence of universal laws and this sets the positivist scientist the task of discovering those laws. The route to achieving this is deemed to be via systematic observation and rational enquiry. However, writers such as Koestler (1964) have questioned the validity of this simple model and emphasized that chance, creativity and even guesswork have an important part to play in the process of scientific discovery. The notion of finding 'universal laws' by a process of painstaking investigation can therefore be seen as an oversimplification.

The notion of a fixed 'universal law' can also be seen to be an oversimplification. It implies that the task of the scientist is to establish certainty. However, this view is disputed by the 'Heisenberg principle':

> This principle relates to the work of Heisenberg (1958) whose study of elementary particles in physics showed that they did not behave exactly as predicted, that some degree of variability or unpredictability always remained. (See Stevens: 1983). On this basis it was argued that some element of doubt or indeterminacy (i.e. uncertainty) is inevitable. The most that can be achieved is probability.
>
> (Thompson 1990b: 38)

One of the basic premises of positivism is therefore seriously challenged by Heisenberg's work. Indeed, within the scientific community, this aspect of positivism holds far less sway than it once did, as Giddens (1993a: 9) confirms: 'the idea that natural science deals only, or even primarily, in law-like generalization belongs to a view of scientific activity which has now largely become abandoned'.

When the idea of 'universal law' is applied to *social* science, its validity becomes even more tenuous. Social science concerns itself with what is distinctively social and therefore encompasses considerable diversity in terms of cultural patterns, economic and political systems and social structures. The concept of 'universal laws' is therefore a very problematic one in this context.

Objectivity

Another major feature of positivism is its insistence on objectivity, in the sense of a clear focus on observable and measurable phenomena with little or no value attached to subjective factors. The strength of this is that it offers considerable rigour by minimizing the scope for subjectivity and rendering propositions testable by experimental means. However, this degree of rigour is not without its costs.

First, by insisting on this criterion of openness to observation, many theoretical approaches which have much to offer as explanatory frameworks are deemed to be invalid on the grounds that their propositions are not empirically testable. However, there is an inherent contradiction in this; the argument that only empirically testable propositions are valid is not itself empirically testable:

> This approach rules out many theoretical/philosophical propositions as invalid science. The scope of theoretical enquiry is therefore severely restricted. Habermas (1972) argues that it is not acceptable as it denies the validity of other epistemologies. If we examine the positivist epistemology we have no way of assessing its validity because it renders untenable any means of investigation other than positivism itself. It therefore places itself in an unassailable position. Positivism cannot evaluate positivism (as such an evaluation would itself not meet the criteria of validity) and no non-positivist critique can be valid as positivism is held to be the only valid method! In short, the logic of positivism is self-contradictory.
>
> (Thompson 1992a: 15)

There is, therefore, a certain amount of dishonesty implicit in the positivist approach to scientific enquiry.

Second, the narrow focus of positivism leaves much of the subject matter of the human services closed to scientific investigation, as they do not fall readily under the spotlight of empirical study:

> Positivism excludes subjective factors without offering a viable alternative; it simply regards them as being inappropriate as an area of study. An approach to social work which neglects the areas of wishes, fears and so on, because they are difficult to measure or verify, is unlikely to be very effective when social work operates where stress and various emotions tend to be at their strongest.
>
> (Thompson 1992a: 15)

The same argument can, of course, be applied to other forms of human services practice, especially health care, as it has long been recognized that health is not simply a (measurable) biological phenomenon, but also depends on a complex web of social, cognitive, perceptual and emotional factors. That is, health has a strong subjective dimension which positivism fails to address.

Value-free science

Positivist science seeks to be objective not only in the sense of 'observable', but also in the sense of being neutral and value-free. As far as social science is concerned, this is a problematic proposition, as we shall see below. However, the situation relating to natural science is similarly problematic, although not so readily recognized as such.

Natural science is often seen as 'real' science, based on rigorous methodology and strictly neutral in its moral and political standpoint. However, this is a gross oversimplification and ignores a significant number of ways in which values influence natural science. These include:

- Sources of funding (for example, government departments, military sources) are likely to operate from a value position which can influence the choice of researcher(s), the nature and parameters of the study and so on.
- The choice of research area, and the particular topic within that area, reflect a set of priorities and therefore values.
- Research is carried out within the context of paradigms and theories. Theories are parts of broader schools of thought (paradigms) and, as we saw in Chapter 2, these are inevitably influenced by values, normative assumptions and ideologies.
- The outcome of research can have major social and political consequences (for example, the use of nuclear energy).

The reality of 'value-free' science is therefore very different from the rhetoric. What is particularly important to note in this respect is that, while these points may be widely accepted within the scientific community, the myth of value-free science continues to hold considerable sway within the popular consciousness, that is, at an

Practice Focus 3.1

Morag completed her BSc in biochemistry and was keen to find a post as a researcher. However, after many failed attempts, she decided to put her knowledge to good use by pursuing a career in nursing. She started a course at the school of nursing attached to the local hospital. Unfortunately, though, this proved to be a big mistake for her.

Morag had been so firmly grounded in 'hard' science that she really struggled to adjust to the holistic perspective of the course. To her, it appeared to be very woolly and lacking in rigour. This problem was intensified when she began her first ward experience. Here she found that the 'swampy lowlands' of practice were not at all in keeping with her way of thinking. The matter very quickly came to a head when she was criticized for her 'impersonal' attitude towards patients and her failure to understand the complexities of working with people. It was at this point that she decided to leave the course and to resume her former plan of pursuing a career in research.

ideological level. The myth therefore remains a very powerful one, particularly for those who are not involved in scientific investigation but who may be influenced by scientific findings – human services staff, for example.

Feyerabend (1975) goes a step further by arguing that science is not only incorrectly characterized as value-free, but is also an actual or potential source of oppression. As Smith (1998: 205) explains:

> Feyerabend developed a standpoint which suggested that science was not rational, that no knowledge rules had operated effectively in any case and that scientific knowledge could be oppressive rather than an instrument of progress . . . For Feyerabend, to treat science as rational and objective enterprise was a myth (that is, folklore for scientists). In addition, he portrayed the pursuit of rational scientific explanations (running from the positivists through to Popper) as undesirable because it substituted the accumulation of knowledge for the goal of emancipating human beings.

The widely accepted notion that science is not only a value-free undertaking but also an entirely positive enterprise for humankind is therefore clearly one that needs to be questioned.

The same points about the myth of value freedom also apply to social science, but with the added dimension of social scientists being part and parcel of the subject matter they study. Because social scientists are part of society, their work cannot become entirely disentangled from the social context of the researchers concerned. This is captured in a classic text of sociology (Aron 1965: 12): 'It is impossible for a study of a given society, however scientific its aims, not to contain implied approval or criticism of that society'. I shall return to this point below.

Empirical research

In keeping with the emphasis on observable phenomena as the basis of valid science, empirical study is seen as the primary foundation of science. However, it has been argued that, while empirical research clearly has an important part to play in knowledge development, its role has tended to be overemphasized. To counterbalance this, it is argued, there is a need to recognize more fully the important role of the *interpretation* of the data generated. As Berger and Kellner (1981: 43) comment:

> There are no 'raw facts' in science; there are only facts within a specific conceptual framework. It is important to see, though, that this can also be said of ordinary life. There too, there are no 'raw facts', but facts embodied in structures of relevance and

> meaning. That is, ordinary life is also organised in the minds of all who participate in it, and this organisation takes place by means of a conceptual framework – however, unsophisticated or illogical this may be, and however dimly the participants may be aware of it.

This relates back to our earlier discussion of informal theory, the use of theoretical frameworks, however informal and 'unofficial' as the basis of making sense of social facts. As is generally made clear on introductory social science courses, the facts do not speak for themselves – they have to be interpreted within a theoretical framework, formal or otherwise. It is this basic premise which positivism, with its zeal for observable phenomena, tends to neglect. It is this which led Winch (1958) to emphasize the need for a stronger focus on making greater sense of what we already know, rather than continuing to produce more and more data. As Shotter (1975: 38) comments:

> And many issues in the social sciences, Winch argues, belong more to philosophy than to science and are, therefore, to be settled by *a priori* conceptual analysis rather than by further empirical research; they are matters of ordering and clarifying what we already know, rather than matters of factual ignorance.

The empirical focus of positivism can therefore produce an imbalance in which what is produced is a great deal of *information*, but relatively little *understanding*. This is particularly problematic for practice-related subjects such as the human services, as I shall argue below with regard to the use and limitations of research.

The distinctiveness of social science

Within social science, positivism manifests itself as a belief in the appropriateness of applying natural science methods and procedures to the study of society. What this fails to take into account is the fundamental differences between nature and society. As Giddens (1993a: 85–6) puts it:

> The difference between the social and natural world is that the latter does not constitute itself as 'meaningful': the meanings it has are produced by human beings in the course of their practical life, and as a consequence of their endeavours to understand or explain it for themselves. Social life – of which these endeavours are a part – on the other hand, is *produced* by its component actors precisely in terms of their active constitution and reconstitution of frames of meaning whereby they organize their experience.

To see social science simply as an extension of natural science is therefore a significant error, as it overlooks a central feature of social life, the fact that social processes and structures are produced or reproduced in and by human action.

A second significant difference is what Giddens (1993a) describes as a 'double hermeneutic'. By this he means a two-way interaction between the knowledge base generated by social science and society itself:

> . . . the double hermeneutic of the social sciences places them in a quite different position to that of natural science in one basic respect. The concepts and theories produced in the natural sciences quite regularly filter into lay discourse and become appropriated as everyday frames of reference. But this is of no relevance, of course, to the world of nature itself; whereas the appropriateness of technical concepts and theories invented by social scientists can turn them into constituting elements of that very 'subject-matter' they were coined to characterize, and by that token *alter* the context of their application.
>
> (Giddens 1993a: 86)

A positivist approach to social science is therefore inappropriate, as it ignores this active dimension of social science – the fact that social scientists and their work are part of the fabric of the society they study, part of the process of creating and recreating that society.

Alternatives to positivism

There are clearly many problems in adopting a positivist approach to the human services. Perhaps the most significant of these is the tendency of the factors outlined above to result in *determinism*, a view of human action as being determined by factors beyond our control. That human action is *conditioned*, or influenced, by external factors is a readily acceptable proposition. However, this is a far cry from the notion that our actions are *determined* by such factors. Such an extreme view, implicit in positivism, has the effect of dehumanizing human subjects, treating us as artefacts of nature, rather than conscious social actors who play an active part in plotting the course of our lives. This raises a number of important issues, some of which will be addressed in Chapter 4.

We need to be careful, though, that we do not 'throw the baby out with the bathwater' by rejecting not only positivist science but science itself. The distorted version of science represented by positivism is referred to as 'scientism'. The question is, therefore: 'Can we reject scientism without also rejecting science?' Giddens (1993b: 20) defines science as:

> . . . the use of systematic methods of investigation, theoretical thinking, and the logical assessment of arguments, to develop a

> body of knowledge about a particular subject-matter. Scientific work depends on a mixture of boldly innovative thought and the marshalling of evidence to support or disconfirm hypotheses and theories. Information and insights accumulated through scientific study and debate are always to some degree *tentative* – open to being revised, or even completely discarded, in the light of new evidence or arguments.

Clearly, research and theory development in the human services can proceed on this basis without making any of the overambitious claims of scientism. There are, therefore, alternatives to positivism, in particular hermeneutical science and critical theory. I shall outline each of these in turn before focusing in particular on some key issues relating to the role of research.

Hermeneutical science

While positivism seeks to exclude the subjective dimension, hermeneutics places subjectivity at centre stage. The objective, external world is meaningless without a subjectivity (a conscious human subject) to interpret it. Thus, for hermeneutical science, the object of study is not the objective world *per se*, but the interrelationship of the objective world with subjective actors who experience it. In fact, the term *experience* is a central one for, as Laing (1967: 20) puts it: 'Theory is the articulated vision of experience'. Behaviour is observed from the outside, while 'experience' refers to what happens within – and it is this internal, experiential dimension which has tended to be neglected in studies of the human services. As Smith (1998: 161) comments: 'hermeneutics focuses upon the lived experience of human beings in their social and historical context'.

In short, hermeneutics is a science of the *person*, focusing on people as active subjects, rather than inert objects, puppets of external forces. This is captured by Shotter (1975: 14) in his quest for a new approach to psychology as a science:

> Thus our problem is: can we construct a human science, just as rigorous and disciplined as a natural science, but which is concerned not with discovering the order and structure of things 'outside' us, but with the order and structure of things 'inside' us, in the intersubjectively shared meanings and understandings by which we live our lives?

Hermeneutical science is therefore a counterbalance to the positivist emphasis on objectivity and it achieves this by reintroducing the subjective or experiential dimension absent from scientism. This makes scientific investigation more difficult and more complex, and a different undertaking from traditional positivist studies. However, this approach can be seen to be more in keeping with the demands of professional practice. As Schön (1992: 53) comments:

> Given the dominant view of professional rigor, the view which prevails in the intellectual climate of the universities and is embedded in the institutional arrangements of professional education and research, rigorous practice depends on well-formed problems of instrumental choice to whose solution research-based theory and technique are applicable. But real-world problems do not come well-formed. They tend to present themselves, on the contrary, as messy, indeterminate, problematic situations.

That is, the reality of practice is far closer to the hermeneutical model of science than it is to the positivist.

Critical theory

The term 'critical theory' is used in two senses, narrow and broad. In its narrow sense, it refers to the work of theorists such as Horkheimer, Marcuse and Habermas (see Jay 1973; Held 1980), who sought to integrate elements of marxism (power, oppression, conflict, social structure) with elements of psychoanalysis (meaning, interpretation, desire). In its broader sense, critical theory refers to a range of theoretical analyses which seek to integrate hermeneutical (or 'phenomenological') issues with wider social or political factors. It is in this second sense that I shall be using it here.

It is also important to note that critical theory is currently a very active and rapidly developing theoretical perspective engaged with issues of 'postmodernism' and the critique of traditional forms of intellectual inquiry and theory building (Lash 1990; Shotter 1993). This topic is discussed below.

Critical theory shares with hermeneutics a dissatisfaction with positivism's neglect of subjective factors. It accepts the basic tenets of hermeneutics but argues that the focus on subjectivity needs to be located in the broader context of society and politics. Although each of us is a unique individual, we also have to take account of the ways in which we are not unique, the commonalities we share with other groups in society and, therefore, the differences between those groups. Critical theory therefore recognizes the importance of subjectivity, but also recognizes that each individual is 'socially located' in terms of class, race, gender and other social divisions. Everitt *et al.* (1992: 20) express this point in the following terms:

> Critical theorists, . . . both Marxists and feminists, would argue that individual interpretations of the world, subjective interpretations, can be understood by reference to the social contexts in which they have been formed. Thus class, gender and race, for

> example, structure the ways in which we experience and make sense of the world. Autonomous creative thought is limited by social structures and processes.

Social science therefore needs to understand not only individual subjectivities but also shared subjectivities in terms of membership of social groups. Critical theory is therefore entirely consistent with anti-discriminatory practice.

Critical theory is often seen as a rebuttal of hermeneutics. However, it can also be seen as an *extension* of hermeneutical science, a development of this approach rather than a rejection of it. Critical theory continues the hermeneutical tradition of acknowledging the significance of experience. It sees subjectivity as a *necessary* condition for understanding human action, but it is not a *sufficient* condition.

Postmodernism

The term 'postmodernism' refers to a broad and complex body of thought which has, in part at least, grown out of poststructuralist thought (Burr 1995). As I have argued previously:

> Postmodernism is not so much a theoretical perspective as a style of theorizing. It encompasses a wide diversity of theoretical positions and political viewpoints.
>
> (Thompson 1998a: 55)

A unifying theme of the postmodernist approach is a rejection of the Enlightenment ideal of humanity marching steadily forward towards a higher and better level as a result of the 'progress' brought about by the development of science and rationality (Smith 1998: 65). Postmodernist thinkers reject as a myth this idea of progress and argue that society has reached, or is about to reach, a period of *post*modernity, in which the assumptions of inevitable progress are breaking down, to be replaced by 'a more sceptical awareness of the limits of human thought and endeavour' (Pugh 1997: 98).

A detailed exposition of postmodernism is certainly beyond the scope of this book. We shall return to the subject of postmodernism in Chapter 4, but one important point to note here is that the emphasis on postmodernist discourses in contemporary social science adds significantly to the critique of positivism and the recognition that an uncritical approach to traditional notions of science is a far from adequate basis for approaching issues relating to the use of formal knowledge in the context of human services practice.

The role of research

The terms 'research' and 'science' are very closely associated, research being seen as the primary tool of scientific investigation. For some, research is very much a positivistic enterprise, as Seaman's (1987: 3) definition shows:

> Scientific research is a process in which observable, verifiable data are systematically collected from the empirical world – the world we know through our senses – in order to describe, explain or predict events. Scientific research differs from non-scientific research undertaken by scholars such as theologians, whose work may be careful and systematic but concerned with unseen phenomena such as supernatural spirits. In contrast, scientific research deals only with what can be observed by one scientist and verified by another.

This passage is highly significant in two ways:

1. It is *wrong*. Much 'scientific' research relates to non-observable phenomena. How many astronomers have 'seen' a black hole?
2. It is *misleading*. The definition draws a distinction between observable phenomena and 'unseen phenomena such as supernatural spirits'. These are two extremes of a very wide continuum, with a considerable amount of scientific research falling in between these two extremes.

It is therefore important to begin our discussion of the role of research in the human services with an explicit acknowledgement that the term 'research' is not being used in this narrow positivist sense. Our concern is with science rather than scientism.

The role of research in relating theory to practice is a complex one and the examination of issues here is therefore far from comprehensive. This subject could easily justify a whole book in its own right. None the less, it is to be hoped that the points raised here can cast at least some light on these issues and thereby contribute to taking forward our understanding.

LoBiondo-Wood and Haber (1990: 5) see research as 'the link between theory, education and practice'. Relating theory to practice can loosely be seen as the application of *knowledge*, particularly formal knowledge, to day-to-day practice. Much of this formal knowledge base can be seen to derive from research findings and the debates which have arisen from them. Practitioners who make explicit use of formal knowledge are therefore *consumers of* research, and practitioners who make implicit use of such knowledge (that is, *all* practitioners) are at least indirect consumers of research.

Formal knowledge to guide practice can derive directly from research studies, for example health care treatment methods or styles of intervention with young people within the youth justice system. That is, certain aspects of the professional knowledge base are strongly research-driven. However, research can also influence practice knowledge more indirectly. For example, the Children Act 1989 is a major basis of formal knowledge within the field of childcare. The Act is, however, heavily dependent on research findings accumulated over a period of many years (Department of Health 1991). Clearly, though, such research was not the only factor in the development of the Children Act 1989 – there were, of course, other, political factors at work also.

However, the role of research is not restricted to that of a source of formal knowledge. It also features as:

- *A justification for practice*: research is often used, appropriately or otherwise, in an attempt to justify a particular course of action or approach – what has come to be known as 'evidence-based practice' (Macdonald *et al.* 1992).
- *The outcome of practice*: much research activity in the human services is based on actual practice (for example, evaluation studies or participant observation).
- *A challenge to theory*: practice can be influenced indirectly by research when the latter poses a challenge to established theory and forces a revision or extension of that theory (for example, by producing data which the theory finds hard to explain).

Research can therefore be seen to interlink with theory and practice in a number of ways. In view of this, research needs to be recognized as a significant part of the process of integrating theory and practice.

Types of research

In order to develop further our understanding of the role of research, it is worth considering, albeit briefly, some of the different types of research which relate to the human services.

A major distinction is between quantitative and qualitative research. Quantitative research is geared towards precise measurement and the identification and analysis of significant variables. Qualitative research is less ambitious in its attempts to achieve precision but covers a wider range of variables. Abbott and Sapsford (1992: x) express the distinction as follows:

> Quantitative research, working in the tradition of the physical sciences, aims at reliable measurement of aspects of a situation and seeks to explain variance in these measures – between groups or over time. Its root model is the experiment . . . with its control group to which treatment is not administered – the argument being if two groups differ *only* in the treatment they have received, then this treatment must be responsible for any

Practice Focus 3.2

The seven members of the multidisciplinary child protection team recognized at one of their team meetings that the field of child protection is a rapidly changing and developing one and they were starting to feel that they were beginning to lose touch with current developments. They had long been aware that child protection is a complex area and that complacency about understanding and expertise is a very real danger.

Consequently, they took the initiative of inviting a lecturer with an interest in child protection to attend a staff development meeting with them to discuss recent research findings and explore their implications for practice. The day proved to be a great success for both the team and the lecturer and established a good baseline for future collaboration. The team gained in confidence and returned to their heavy workload with a renewed vigour.

> differences between them. Qualitative researchers, on the other hand, are credited with an holistic approach, refusing to dissect the situation into measurable 'variables', and with the kind of attention to naturalism (studying the situation as it really occurs, not as it seems when modified by the research procedures) which would rule out 'treatments' or control groups.

Some research purists regard qualitative methods as inferior to quantitative ones, and less 'scientific'. However, a more constructive approach is to see the two sets of methods as alternatives to be chosen according to the circumstances. That is, quantitative methods will suit certain situations while qualitative methods will suit others – and, indeed, deciding which are appropriate is a key research skill.

Another important distinction is that between inductive and deductive methods. The former refers to broad 'scans' of data sets to detect significant patterns, structures and commonalities. Deductive research, by contrast, involves the testing of hypotheses, that is measuring theoretical propositions against the findings of empirical studies. However, what is often not fully appreciated is that the two types rarely, if ever, exist in their pure form. For example, within deductive research, there is inevitably an element of inductive reasoning in so far as hypotheses do not appear from nowhere – they arise from a process of induction.

Research can also be classified according to the intended purpose or use of the research outcomes. That is, a distinction is drawn between *pure* and *applied* research. The former refers to research geared towards extending knowledge without a specific practical outcome in mind, whereas the latter is designed in an attempt to produce just such a practical outcome, for example an improvement in policy or professional practice.

The two types of research, though, are not entirely separate. Today's applied research often owes much to yesterday's pure research, in the sense that pure research can raise our level of knowledge and understanding to the point where applied research becomes possible. Pure research is seen by many people as an academic irrelevance, a luxury we cannot afford, unlike the 'pragmatic' basis of applied research. What such a view fails to realize is that the absence of an immediate practical application cannot be equated with the absence of practical value in the long term.

A further type of research, and one becoming increasingly common in the human services, is *evaluative* research. This is a particular form of applied research which seeks to measure the effectiveness of specific policies or interventions. This involves finding a systematic means of measuring progress towards identified objectives. The twofold appeal of this type of research lies in its cost-effectiveness (it is often used as a means of promoting 'value for money' in terms of efficiency and effectiveness) and its value as the basis of professional development – a springboard from which to improve practice and develop skills.

Research criteria

Another aspect of research which needs to be appreciated is the set of criteria by which research is judged. I shall therefore comment briefly on each of the main criteria generally used within the scientific community.

Validity

For research to be valid, the researcher needs to ensure that the instruments used for data collection are appropriate to the task at hand. Gilbert (1993: 27–8) uses the measurement of alcohol as an example:

> For instance, suppose that you want to measure people's consumption of alcohol (a concept). You choose to do this by using a questionnaire in which you will ask respondents to tell you how much they drank during the previous month. In fact, this is not a good indicator of alcohol consumption. People tend to under-report consumption – they say they drink less than they actually drink – casting doubts on the validity of the indicator.

Reliability

A 'reliable' research study is one in which the measurements used are internally consistent. Shipman (1988: ix) captures this point as follows:

> *If the investigation had been carried out again, by different researchers, using the same methods, would the same results have been obtained?* The concern here is with the RELIABILITY of the methods used. This includes not only the way information has been collected, but the dependability of the researcher and the response of those studied.

Rigour

This implies adopting a disciplined and systematic approach to the process of investigation and analysis. It involves adopting what Abbott and Sapsford (1992: 1) call the 'research stance':

> The major difference between the research stance and that of everyday common sense is that good research is always *disciplined* in a way and to an extent which is seldom (unfortunately) typical of our everyday judgements.

Objectivity

It was noted earlier that objective truth, in the sense of independent, value-free science, is an unrealistic goal to aim for. However, Giddens (1993b: 21) argues that sociology (and, by extension, the other social sciences) can be 'objective' in the sense of being open to public scrutiny:

> Objectivity in sociology is thus achieved substantially through the effects of mutual *criticism* by members of the sociological community. Many of the subjects studied in sociology are controversial, because they directly concern disputes and struggles in society itself. But through public debate, the examination of evidence and the logical structure of argument, such issues can be fruitfully and effectively analysed (Habermas, 1979).

This type of objectivity is also often referred to as 'openness' in so far as the basic premises of the research – the process, rationale and outcomes – are open to critical enquiry.

Explanatory power

This refers to the extent to which the research casts new light on the subject under investigation – the degree to which it produces new knowledge or understanding.

The limitations of research

Proponents of research understandably promote the value and benefit of research. However, where the focus is on applying knowledge to practice, rather than simply *developing* knowledge, we must also be careful to recognize the limitations of research. Space does not permit a detailed analysis of these issues, but they are none the less worth exploring in outline at least. I shall focus on five particular areas in which limitations on research can be identified:

1. *Explanatory power versus validity*. Positivist science places heavy stress on validity. One consequence of this is that a relatively small amount of knowledge is produced but with a high level of validity. Other forms of research (for example, participant observation) tend to have lower levels of validity – there is a greater chance of error – but far greater explanatory power. There is, therefore, an inevitable 'trade-off' between validity and explanatory power.

   Because human services work operates at the intersection of psychological, social and political forces, a positivist approach premised on high validity has little to offer. Approaches offering greater explanatory power, however, are more suited to the pragmatic basis of professional practice where a greater range of knowledge is called for. This 'trade-off' between explanatory power and validity therefore acts as a constraint or limitation on the role of research in the human services.
2. *The tentative nature of research*. Our investigations are always open to question and challenge, whether by theoretical analysis or further research which produces contradictory findings. Realistically, we can never say that we have definitively completed our knowledge base in a particular area. We can only say that this is the current extent of our knowledge, the best explanation we can offer to date. That is, what research offers is always *tentative* – probable, but rarely, if ever, definitive.
3. *The sociopolitical context*. As noted earlier, research activity inevitably takes place within a social and political context. This can place considerable limitations on the part research can play in influencing or informing policy and practice. For example, as a result of political forces, attempts may be made to suppress certain research results, as in the case of the Black Report on health inequalities (Townsend and Davidson 1987). Similarly, proposals for research projects have to fall within certain broad social and political parameters if they are to be successful in their bid for funding.
4. *The changing field*. Research produces new information and know-ledge by the very process of investigation. However, as soon as new information is produced, it becomes 'old' information in the sense that it is a snapshot of a moving picture. The subject matter of

the research – policy, practice and related issues in the human services – continues to change and develop beyond the completion of the research. This is a hallmark of social science – that studies and findings need to be reviewed so that their relevance to a changing society can be re-evaluated. For example, valid research findings in one decade may no longer be valid in the following decade due to the changing field to which it relates.

5. *Research as a source of oppression.* Oliver (1992) argues that research in the field of disability studies tends to present disabled people as an *object* of study, and thereby dehumanizes and oppresses them. Similarly, Ramazanoglu (1989: 440) argues that traditional social science practices can be seen as 'creating and legitimating aspects of the oppression of women'. She comments that: 'The objectivity and rigour of western science and social science rests on unreasonable assumptions about the superiority of reason and the associated superiority of men' (1989: 438; see also Harding 1987). Research can therefore have oppressive consequences if issues of power, inequality and social division are not appreciated. This potential for oppression is therefore a significant limitation on the scope of research.

These five examples illustrate the central point that, while research has considerable potential for informing and enhancing both theory and practice, it also has serious limitations in terms of how far it can take us in developing our knowledge and understanding. This is an important point, and one to which we shall return in Chapter 4, where the role of philosophy is examined.

Conclusion: research-minded practice

The term 'science' is one which is often used loosely and uncritically. What we have seen in this chapter is that science, in the positivist sense of the word, is not an appropriate basis for informing professional practice in the human services. As Everitt *et al.* (1992: 62) comment: 'One of the problems about positivism is that the research endeavour is mystified: esoteric skills and techniques serve the interests of the powerful'.

Similarly, Abbott and Sapsford (1992: 3) comment on the mystique of research:

> 'Research' is often presented as something beyond the capability of those who have not undergone long training. It is what is done by scientists, it requires the use of computers and abstruse mathematics, and ordinary untrained people sometimes cannot understand the questions, let alone the answers.

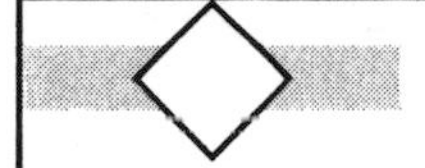

Practice Focus 3.3

Catherine was pleased to have the opportunity to undertake a small-scale research project as part of her professional training. She decided to interview a number of people who regularly attended a psychiatric day centre to gauge their views about the psychiatric services they had received or were receiving.

The project began very well and Catherine was confident it would be a success. However, in one particular interview, the service user became very agitated because she felt Catherine's line of questioning to be very intrusive. This created a lot of tension in the group and made subsequent interviews quite fraught and difficult. In fact, it soon became necessary to abandon the project, as it was causing a great deal of ill-feeling as a result of the mistrust created by the earlier incident.

The mystique of scientism is therefore a disincentive to staff getting involved in research and using it as a tool for improving practice. It creates unnecessary barriers to the development of a professional knowledge base in touch with the realities of day-to-day practice.

However, as we have also seen in this chapter, positivist science is not the only type of science. Research and theory development can be rigorous and systematic without falling foul of the distortions inherent in positivism. We can develop what Shotter (1975: 23) describes as a '*moral science of action* rather than a *natural science of behaviour*'.

Everitt *et al.* (1992: 4) introduce the concept of 'research-minded practice', a notion which is both consistent with, and supportive of, the development of a non-positivist research base:

> Research-minded practice is concerned with the analytical assessment of social need and resources, and the development, implementation and evaluation of strategies to meet that need . . . The taken-for-granted becomes subject to critical scrutiny. An examination of research methodology and exploration of research methods is fundamental to such practice.

Research-minded practice is, as Everitt *et al.* go on to say, *good* practice. It is a positive basis for integrating theory, research and practice, thereby contributing to an informed practice and a theory base which is not divorced from the demands of practice. Everitt *et al.* outline what is involved in research-minded practice and this provides a good starting point for practitioners who recognize the value of developing such an approach.

Thus, research-minded practitioners:

- will be constantly defining and making explicit their objectives and hypotheses;
- will treat their explanations of the social world as hypotheses – that is, as tentative and open to be tested against evidence;
- will be aware of their expertise and knowledge and that of others;
- will bring to the fore theories that help make sense of social need, resources and assist in decision making with regard to strategies;
- will be thoughtful, reflecting on data and theory and contributing to their development and refinement;
- will scrutinise and be analytical of available data and information;
- will be mindful of the pervasiveness of ideology and values in the way we see and understand the world.

(Everitt *et al.* 1992: 4–5)

Research-minded practice reflects a balance, a helpful and constructive midpoint on a continuum which has the rejection of research at one extreme, and an uncritical acceptance of the research findings of 'experts' at the other. Science and research have a valuable contribution to make to the integration of theory and practice in the human services. Research-minded practice is a useful term which succeeds in capturing the important blend of intellectual inquiry and pragmatic application which I shall be proposing as the basis of optimal practice. Research-minded practice is therefore a concept which will reappear in later chapters.

Food for thought

- Consider the concept of 'science'.
  - In what ways can working with people and their problems be described as 'scientific'?
  - What role does social science play in influencing practice in the human services?
  - How could you use a hermeneutical approach in your work?
- Consider the concept of research.
  - What role can or should research play in shaping policy and practice?
  - What is meant by using research *critically*?
  - What are the limitations of research?
- Consider 'research-minded practice'.
  - What does this term mean to you?
  - How could you develop it in your own practice?
  - What barriers to developing it do you think you might encounter?

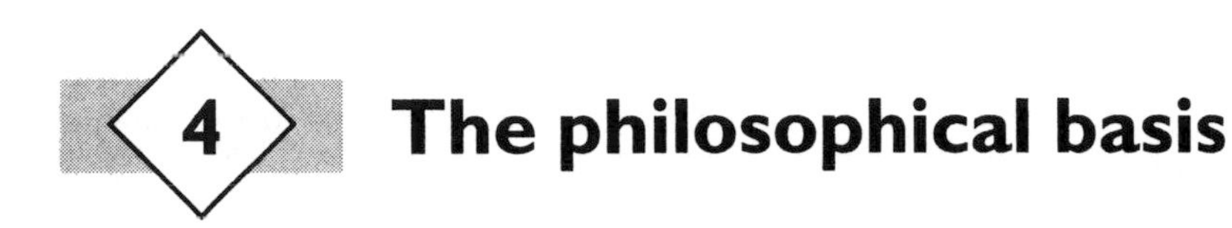

4 The philosophical basis

Chapter overview

- What is philosophy?
- Why is it important?
- Why do we need more than 'eclecticism'?
- What is existentialism?
- How does it relate to human services practice?

Introduction

'Philosophy' is a term which conjures up a number of images which can act as barriers to understanding and using philosophy as a basis for informing and enhancing professional practice. Philosophy is often seen as:

- *Elitist*: it is perceived as a matter reserved for an ivory-tower minority and is not for more general consumption.
- *Difficult*: many aspects of philosophy are difficult. By their very nature, many elements of philosophy are subtle, complex and intricate. However, this is often allowed to mask the fact that many aspects of philosophy are readily understandable.
- *Obscure*: philosophy is commonly regarded as irrelevant to everyday life, an activity which focuses on obscure matters distanced from day-to-day experience.
- *Abstract*: clearly, in some ways philosophy is abstract. It seeks to raise our level of understanding and so some degree of abstraction is inevitable. However, the fact that much philosophy is abstract does not mean that it has no concrete implications or consequences.

One of the primary aims of this chapter is to go some way towards challenging these perceptions and presenting philosophy as an important and valuable tool in facilitating the process of integrating theory and practice. I shall begin by addressing the fundamental question of 'What is philosophy?'

What is philosophy?

The literal meaning of philosophy is 'love of wisdom'. It is used, however, in a number of related senses. It refers to the academic discipline of philosophy, involving the study of the works of established philosophers, ranging from Plato, Aristotle and Socrates to de Beauvoir, Derrida and Foucault. However, it is also used in a much narrower sense to refer to a set of values and beliefs relating to a particular individual group or activity. For example, a group of staff may develop a 'team philosophy', or an organization may wish to publicize its 'training philosophy'.

These two senses of the word 'philosophy', both broad and narrow, can be seen to represent the extremes of a continuum, and there are, of course, other points between the two extremes. For example, any discussion which addresses values or questions existing attitudes or practices may, at times, be termed 'philosophical'.

Unfortunately, the term philosophy has the connotation, for many people at least, of being unconnected with everyday life – an abstraction separate from concrete reality. Philosophy is 'often identified with high-brow ideas irrelevant to the real world and expressed in elitist jargon' (Thompson 1992a: 1). This is particularly unfortunate with regard to integrating theory and practice, as such a negative connotation is likely to widen the gap between the two, rather than facilitate their integration. It is for this reason that the philosophical basis is addressed in this chapter – to dispel some of the misconceptions about philosophy and to clarify the positive role it can play in facilitating high standards of professional practice. An important point to recognize, and clarify, is the overlap between theory and philosophy. The two concepts have much in common but are also significantly different in some respects. Philosophy is like theory in so far as it provides frameworks for explaining and understanding aspects of the world or of our experience. In this respect, philosophy is a type or subdivision of theory. However, it is also more than theory. This applies in terms of the role of values. Theories, particularly those that aspire to 'scientific' status, often attempt to minimize the role of values, whereas a philosophy incorporates values, often as an explicit basis of that philosophy:

> . . . theories attempt to exclude values as far as possible in order to achieve 'scientific' status. A philosophy, by contrast, does not shy

> away from values, it declares them and makes constructive use of them as the basis of a moral philosophy. Ethics is a dimension generally absent from scientific theories but often a key element within a philosophical system. A philosophy is broader than a theory, it is a way of life or window on the world – a 'Weltanschauung'. Values are obviously a key part of such a world view.
>
> (Thompson 1992a: 21)

The notion of *Weltanschauung* is an important one to which I shall return below when existentialist philosophy is discussed. The significance of values, however, is a more immediate concern. As was noted in Chapter 1, values are an integral part of the human services. Any attempt to develop a theoretical basis for professional practice must therefore take account of the role of values. That is, a philosophical perspective is called for.

In Chapter 3, the tension between validity and explanatory power was identified. While positivism concentrates on the former, hermeneutical science concentrates on the latter. Similarly, philosophy places great value on explanatory power and seeks validity not from empirical rigour, but from the strength of its arguments. This focus on explanatory power gives philosophy a higher degree of applicability to practice than a narrower, more technical theoretical approach. A greater willingness to tackle value issues makes philosophy of greater relevance, potentially at least, to the needs and concerns of practitioners.

This point relates closely to Schön's (1983) critique of 'technical rationality' as the basis of professional practice. He argues that the technical rationality of science is well-suited to clearly defined, well-bounded problems but lacks the flexibility to deal with the indeterminacy and 'messiness' of the problems encountered in professional practice. He writes of the 'dilemma of rigor or relevance', which has much in common with the validity versus explanatory power distinction discussed above. Technical rationality may produce a rigorous knowledge base but it will have limited relevance to the world of day-to-day practice:

> This dilemma of 'rigor or relevance' arises more acutely in some areas of practice than others. In the varied topography of professional practice, there is a high, hard ground where practitioners can make effective use of research-based theory and technique, and there is a swampy lowland where situations are confusing 'messes' incapable of technical solution. The difficulty is that the problems of the high ground, however great their technical interest, are often relatively unimportant to clients or to the larger society, while in the swamp are the problems of

> greatest human concern. Shall the practitioner stay on the high, hard ground where he can practice rigorously, as he understands rigor, but where he is constrained to deal with problems of relatively little social importance? Or shall he descend to the swamp where he can engage the most important and challenging problems if he is willing to forsake technical rigor?
>
> (Schön 1983: 42)

Schön uses the term 'artistry' to describe the skills and knowledge used in an almost intuitive way in addition to, or as a counterbalance to, the technical rationality of science. In short, he sees professional practice as a combination of art and science.

An important aspect of Schön's distinction between the high ground of science and the lowland of practice is the need to see problem-solving in the context of 'problem-setting'. Professional practice is concerned with problem-solving. However, what is not so fully recognized is the process of problem-setting – the process by which a problem and its parameters are defined and interpreted. In general, there is relatively little attention paid to the 'swampy' process of problem-setting, while the 'technical rationality' of theory and research has tended to concentrate on finding solutions to the problems. It is not without significance that:

1. Technical rationality is better suited to accounting for problem-solving than problem-setting. This is consistent with the discussion in Chapter 3 of 'problematics'. A theory or paradigm will tend to focus on the problematic it can best explain.
2. A central factor in the process of problem-setting is that of values. How a situation becomes defined as a problem will depend, to a large extent, on value judgements. The values of the people involved in problem-setting will be very influential in determining what is unacceptable in a situation – and therefore in what way it constitutes a problem.

Although Schön does not explicitly advocate a philosophical approach, his critique of technical rationality does pave the way for a greater emphasis on philosophy, particularly, as we shall see below, on certain types of philosophy.

A further way in which philosophy can be seen to go beyond theory is in terms of its capacity to operate at a 'metatheoretical' level. That is, a philosophy can integrate a number of theories by providing an overview, an overarching framework which provides a more holistic perspective than individual theories. In this way, philosophy overlaps with the notion of 'Grand Theory' discussed in Chapter 2.

Human services work is underpinned by a variety of theoretical perspectives. These theoretical strands sometimes overlap but are often incompatible or contradictory. Philosophy is capable of combining disparate concepts into a coherent framework. Traditionally, such a combining of elements is known as 'eclecticism'. However, the philosophical approach I am proposing here is significantly different from eclecticism, as I shall make clear in the following section.

Beyond eclecticism

The term 'eclectic' is frequently used to describe an approach to practice which incorporates a range of theoretical concepts, themes and issues. However, as I have argued previously, the uncritical linking together of diverse theoretical components has dubious validity as the basis of an informed approach to practice:

> Eclecticism fails because it juxtaposes incompatible theories without placing them within the context of a conceptual framework which uses higher order concepts (such as paradox) to make sense of the combination. In other words, instead of *linking* theories together, eclecticism simply *lumps* them together.
>
> (Thompson 1992a: 21–2)

To describe one's theoretical perspective as 'eclectic' can be a simple avoidance of addressing the complex and thorny issues of the relationship between theory and practice. It is an example of *reductionism* in so far as it reduces a complex question to a simple answer.

The strength of eclecticism is that it allows practitioners to draw on a wide range of ideas, techniques and methods and encourages, to a certain extent at least, a cross-fertilization of ideas and thus the development of new approaches. However, what also needs to be recognized is the major disadvantage of a lack of coherence and structure. Eclecticism is the equivalent of placing alongside each other the components of a machine, and expecting the machine to work, without any attempt to link the components together in any logical or coherent way. Or, to use a different analogy, eclecticism is 'a simple juxtaposition of incompatible elements – all the ingredients of an excellent dish but no recipe' (Thompson 1992a: 177). Eclecticism is the term we use for jumbling together a range of concepts and techniques without considering how they interrelate with one another, or whether they are compatible. In adopting an eclectic approach, we treat ideas as individual tools, rather than cogs or components of a wider system. In this way, eclecticism holds back the development of our thinking and practice. We may add an extra tool here or there, but eclecticism can offer little more.

However, we should be careful not to confuse rejecting a simple eclecticism with a rejection of the possibility of combining elements from different theoretical perspectives. It *is* possible to make such links, but this needs to be done at a metatheoretical or *philosophical* level. That is, instead of simply viewing one theory from the perspective of another, we need to obtain an overview of two or more theories, to rise above the level of technical theory – hence the term *meta*theoretical. In order to achieve this, we need to adopt a particular type of reasoning, a mode of thought which allows and facilitates the synthesis of disparate elements. It is to this that we now turn.

Dialectical reason

Conventional logic is *analytical*. That is, it involves breaking situations down into their component parts so that a complex matter can be understood in simpler terms. Such an analysis, by its very nature, produces a snapshot rather than a moving picture. It is therefore ill-equipped to account for conflict, change and development. For this reason, it is necessary to consider an alternative form of reasoning, namely *dialectical* reason.

Dialectical reason does not contradict or invalidate analytical reason – it goes beyond it. Analytical reason breaks things down into their component parts, and this is an essential first step in the process of understanding. It is, however, only a first step and needs to be followed by *synthesis* – the linking together of those parts into a coherent whole. This process of synthesis, or as I shall call it below 'totalization', is the hallmark of dialectical reason:

> Dialectical reason incorporates analytical logic but transcends it. It breaks things down into component parts but this is not sufficient. It then goes on to synthesise them into a concrete whole. It overcomes the danger of being 'abstract', that is, of taking a partial view and proclaiming it to be the whole. For example, behaviourism takes one aspect of psychology – learning theory – and presents it as the whole truth. Analysis is only the first step and synthesis must follow.
>
> (Thompson 1992a: 51)

The basis of dialectical reason is conflict. The dialectic refers to the process by which conflicting forces come together and produce change. This process is perhaps best known in relation to marxism, as indicated by the term 'dialectical materialism'.

The process, in its simplest form, can be seen to work as follows: A particular force (the thesis) enters into conflict with another force (the antithesis) and, as a result of this interaction of conflicting forces, a new situation is produced (the synthesis). It is in this way that dialectical reason is cyclical – the synthesis becomes a new thesis and thus enters into conflict with a new antithesis, thus producing a new cycle of dialectical change. For marxism, the dialectic is the primary means by which we can understand history (although Marx himself did not express this directly in terms of thesis-antithesis-synthesis; McLellan 1975).

This model can be seen to apply to interpersonal dynamics in which two or more people enter into conflict over a certain issue or set of issues, and from this a new position or understanding is achieved (a synthesis). However, this may then prove to be the basis of further conflicts of interest or perspective – and thus the basis of a new cycle of the dialectic.

Dialectical reason can therefore be seen to have two advantages over analytical reason:

1. *It can more easily account for conflict.* Indeed, it recognizes the central role of conflict of interests as a factor in social life.
2. *It can account for change.* That is, it is dynamic, rather than static. As such, it avoids the pitfall of presenting a 'snapshot' which can very quickly become out of date.

A further important advantage of dialectical reason is its ability to clarify the relationship between the individual and society, a very important consideration as far as both social work and health care are concerned. As we have seen, the notion of 'synthesis' is a central one to dialectical reason. Sartre (1976) uses the term 'totalization' to refer to the same process. He sees the interaction of the individual and society as a dialectical process of totalization, a dialectic of subjectivity and objectivity.

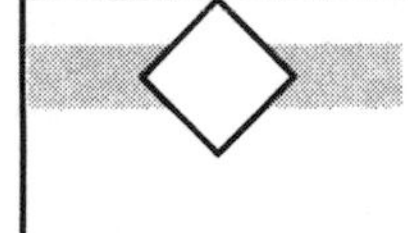

Practice Focus 4.1

Tim and Wendy both joined the team at the same time and it was immediately apparent that sparks were going to fly as their approaches to the work were poles apart and each showed little tolerance for the opposing view. This led to some 'colourful' discussions between the two and a constant tension brought about by the inherent conflict.

Over time, however, it became clear that they were learning from each other and, although they were never going to see eye-to-eye, they became accommodated to one another. This was to prove to be important for, when a proposed reorganization threatened to break up the team, Wendy and Tim joined forces to become a very powerful force in challenging the proposal. In effect, the conflict between the two staff was now entering a new phase of the dialectic, a new stage in a process of change premised on the interaction of conflicting forces.

The individual's experience of the world is, of course, subjective. However, the individual is constrained by external social forces. In this way, the subjective life-world of the individual enters into conflict with the objective world of social and political forces. Thus, a further 'totalization' takes place as the individual interacts with the social world. Simply living our daily lives can therefore be seen as a process of dialectical totalization. Berger and Luckmann (1966: 149) comment as follows:

> Since society exists as both objective and subjective reality any adequate theoretical understanding of it must comprehend both these aspects ... The individual member of society ... simultaneously externalizes it as an objective reality. In other words, to be in society is to participate in its dialectic.

Clearly, this is a complex area of study but, none the less, an important one for casting light on significant aspects of our experience of the human services. In order to develop our understanding of dialectical reason, and the major part it can play in integrating theory and practice, I shall look in more detail at a particular philosophy which makes explicit use of dialectical reason – that of existentialism. However, before presenting an account of existentialism, it is important to stress that, although I am presenting existentialism as a particularly useful approach to the human services, it is by no means the only one. It is an example of *a* philosophical approach, rather than *the* philosophical approach. The work of Foucault (1977, 1979) also raises a number of issues relevant to the human services (Abbott and Sapsford 1988; Rojek *et al.* 1988) as does the development of postmodernist thought in general. I shall therefore make relatively brief comment on the role of postmodernism as one example of a philosophical approach before addressing the main topic of existentialism in far more detail.

Postmodernism

As we noted in Chapter 3, postmodernism is a broad theoretical approach. It would be hopelessly unrealistic to attempt to provide a detailed analysis of its import as a contribution to contemporary philosophical thought. I shall therefore restrict myself to comments on a small number of postmodernist themes and signal their relevance for the integration of theory and practice.

Fragmentation

Critical of the 'grand theory' approach, postmodernists argue that social reality is characterized more by *fragmentation* than by any unified or integrated whole (Carter 1998). They reject the traditional emphasis on 'universalization' (looking for universal truths – an activity postmodernists disparagingly refer to as 'foundationalism') and 'totalization' (the development of an overarching framework or 'metanarrative'). Postmodernists are far less ambitious in their expectations of what theory and academic inquiry can achieve and are therefore sceptical of many of the claims of traditional theorists.

Postmodernism presents social reality as far more complex and fragmentary than is generally recognized in other approaches to the study of social life. The expectation that theory can provide relatively simple formulations for understanding social reality or simple solutions is therefore one that finds no space within postmodernist thought.

Logocentrism

Fox (1993: 8) explains logocentrism in the following terms:

> In scientific discourse, logocentrism inheres in the claim that scientific method makes reality accessible, without the intervention of any mediating process which might distort our perception.

Postmodernism rejects logocentrism and argues that reality is not 'given' in any direct sense, but has to be constructed through language and discourse. Great emphasis is therefore placed on the absence of one underlying absolute truth: theory-building is therefore not a matter of looking for 'the truth'. As Hollinger (1994: 174) comments:

> Theory is thus important to postmodernists, but the task of theory, and its basic orientation, is not the universal truth of the Enlightenment but specific to the demands of the day. One must be more rigorous and honest than defenders of the dogmas of the Enlightenment can allow themselves to be; we need to examine our questions and assumptions critically and test their limits.

Différance

This is a term used by Derrida (1976) to describe the 'slippery' quality of social reality as a result of the absence of hard and fast 'answers' and the impact of constant change. It arises from the complexities of language and meaning. As Fox (1993: 7–8) puts it:

> *Différance* is inevitable once one enters into a language or other symbolic mode of representation, in which signifiers can refer not to referents (the 'underlying reality'), but only to other signifiers. While trying to represent the real, one finds that the meaning that one is trying to communicate slips from one's grasp.

> We are left not with the reality, but with an approximation which, however much we try to make it 'more real', is always already deferred and irrecoverable.

It is perhaps ironic (and also typically postmodernist) that this passage is in itself an example of what it describes: the difficulty in 'grasping' reality in any direct sense. In terms of the relationship between theory and practice, of course, this is very significant, as it means that theory can never quite 'catch up' with practice, that there will always be a gap between the two because of these difficulties in 'pinning down' the slippery nature of social reality.

Affirmation of diversity

Difference is a key term in the postmodernist vocabulary: 'difference is seen as being in opposition to normalization, the tendency to attempt to impose restrictive social norms at the expense of diversity and heterogeneity' (Thompson 1998a: 61). Postmodernist thought is therefore supportive of the notion of social diversity and the value of recognizing the significant differences between individuals and between groups of people. Best and Kellner (1991) link this to the notion of a 'politics of difference', recognizing that the denial of difference is a means of maintaining the political *status quo* and thus perpetuating inequality and forms of oppression. In this respect, postmodernism is consistent with the value base of anti-discriminatory practice, although this is not always the case as far as postmodernist writers are concerned (see Boyne and Rattansi 1990).

The broad philosophical movement of postmodernism has challenged a great deal of traditional theory and raised a number of important questions. This critical perspective on traditional theory is something that is shared with another broad philosophical movement – that of existentialism – and it is to this that we now turn.

Existentialism

There are a number of texts which explore aspects of the relationship between nursing and philosophy (Gray and Pratt 1990), and between social work and philosophy (Timms and Watson 1976, 1978). Such texts tend to promote the view that philosophy has a part to play in guiding human services practice. However, while the view that philosophy *per se* has much to offer has been presented, what also needs to be taken into account is the value of *specific* philosophies. Space does not permit a detailed discussion of a range of philosophical perspectives and so I shall be concentrating on existentialism, a philosophy which offers considerable explanatory power with regard to issues of the human services.

Existentialism is one example of a holistic philosophy which has had some impact on counselling and psychotherapy, especially in the USA (May *et al.* 1958; Frankl 1973), but a very limited impact on social work (although not quite so limited in the USA; see, for example, Stretch 1967; Krill 1978).

Existentialism offers a 'philosophy of existence', a conceptual framework which aims to understand human existence in terms of freedom and responsibility, and the problems and complexities we encounter when we exercise such freedom (in the form of choices and decisions) and take responsibility for the consequences of our actions. It seeks to locate such freedom (the fundamental freedom of being responsible for ourselves) in the wider social context of the structure of society, in terms of social constraints and influences, for example class (Sartre 1976), race/ethnicity (Sartre 1948), gender (de Beauvoir 1972) or age (Thompson 1995a, 1998b).

Existentialism emphasizes the dialectical interaction of individual factors (my choices, values, actions) and wider sociopolitical factors (the oppressions of sexism and racism). It is not a case of working out which dimension is more important, the personal or the social, but rather a matter of understanding existence as a constant interplay of the two, a dynamic process simultaneously personal and social.

Existentialism can therefore be a helpful philosophy when it comes to making sense of some of the complexities of discrimination and oppression and their significant role in the human services (Thompson 1998c). As Birt (1997: 206) comments:

> The various forms of social oppression and domination obstruct the actualization of that freedom which constitutes the being of human reality, thereby blocking the ultimate source of energy for the creative formation of identity. Thus, oppression may be seen as an existential violation, an ontological crime. Is this not what is meant when we describe oppression and exploitation as de-humanizing?

Existentialism has been shown to offer a firm basis for developing a holistic and pragmatic theory base for social work (Thompson 1992a, 1992b), and the arguments could similarly be extended to account for the human services more broadly.

A central concern of existentialism is that of *ontology*, the study of being. Fundamental questions about the nature and purpose of existence can make us feel very uncomfortable, and so we often disregard such issues without facing up to them. However, there are times when it is difficult not to face up to such matters: At times of crisis, the

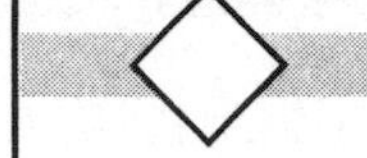

Practice Focus 4.2

Pat was an experienced health visitor who enrolled on a specialist course relating to the care of older people. On the course she was introduced to the concept of ageism and the social and political factors associated with old age. At first she found these ideas very unsettling, as they seemed to undermine everything she had learned about older people and did not fit with her experience. She had been taught to see each patient as a unique individual and to focus very much on the personal, individual level. Now older people were being presented from a very different perspective with a strong emphasis on old age as a sociological matter.

As the course continued, though, she became more comfortable with the sociological perspective and came to realize that what she was learning served to complement her understanding of the individual, rather than to deny it. That is, she appreciated that the experience of older people is both personal and social, and she did not have to abandon one perspective in favour of the other.

stability and equilibrium of our lives ('homeostasis') break down and may leave us in a vulnerable state of confusion:

> As a rule, questions about the purpose and meaning of life are rarely addressed. Within the complacency of homeostasis we take such matters for granted and, if they do arise, they are usually dismissed by jokes about 'the meaning of life' etc. However, at a time of crisis, such issues loom large. Feelings of loneliness, emptiness and meaninglessness are characteristic of crisis as it is, in effect, an existential experience insofar as it replaces the security of homeostasis with doubt and existential uncertainty.
>
> (Thompson 1991b: 17)

The significant point to note here is that the point of intervention in the lives of families and individuals by human services professionals is so often a point of crisis – a time when people's normal coping responses have broken down. There is therefore a danger that workers who have little or no awareness of ontological issues will lack sensitivity in their dealings with service users for whom ontological issues currently have considerable significance as, for example, in situations where:

- grief, loss and bereavement are to the fore;
- depression is a significant feature;
- terminal illness is present;

- life-threatening or near-death experiences have been encountered;
- people's values and beliefs have been challenged or undermined.

Clearly, this covers a wide range of situations which human services staff encounter as part of their professional duties. Ontology is therefore an important facet of the circumstances commonly encountered by human services professionals. Adopting a 'common sense' approach which dismisses or marginalizes ontology is therefore likely to leave staff ill-equipped to deal with some of the most demanding aspects of their work.

Being reluctant to address issues of ontology can, in itself, be explained by ontology, through the concept of *bad faith*. As Barnes (1974: 6) comments: 'Essentially, bad faith is a lie to oneself which rests on the denial that a human being is a free self-making process'. This is a central theme of existentialist philosophy – the notion that we act in bad faith when we try to deny that we are responsible for our own actions, when we draw on a range of excuses to avoid facing up to our freedom. These 'excuses' include:

- *Predetermination*. For example, a man refusing to take ownership of his own sexist behaviour may seek to justify himself by arguing that: 'It was never intended that women should be like men'. Commonly, the word 'natural' is used in an attempt to justify such attitudes: 'It is natural that . . .'.
- *Fixed personality*. Comments like 'I can't help it, that's the way I

Practice Focus 4.3

Lisa was a family centre worker with two years' experience. During that time she had encountered a wide range of problems and demanding situations. However, what she had not encountered during that time was death.

Christopher was a two-year-old who regularly attended the centre with his mother. Christopher was diagnosed shortly after birth as having a degenerative heart condition and so it was known that his life-span could be short. However, knowing this did not make it any easier to cope with the grief when he died a week before his third birthday. Lisa, in particular, was devastated by the loss. She had never experienced the loss of a relative or friend and had never attended a funeral. She had never thought about death or how she would cope with bereavement – she considered such matters 'morbid'. Consequently, she was totally ill-equipped to deal with her feelings. The fact that she was expected to support others, including Christopher's mother, through this difficult period made the situation unbearable, leading to her taking sick-leave for almost three weeks.

am' are similarly used to deny ownership of one's actions. In this way, our own behaviour is presented as being beyond our control because of an ingrained personality structure which 'makes' us behave in a certain way.

- *Biology*. Oppressive behaviour is often legitimized by reference to biological factors. Racism, sexism, ageism and disablism all rely on attempts at justification premised on biological (or pseudo-biological) notions of superiority (Thompson 1998a).
- *Religion*. Certain attitudes or actions are sometimes presented as being beyond an individual's control on religious grounds. For example, some people may claim that they had no choice behaving in a particular way because it was 'God's will'.
- *Behaviourism*. Some forms of behavioural psychology deny the existence of free will and regard behaviour as the outcome of 'behavioural contingencies' (conditioning, reinforcement and so on). This again presents behaviour as emanating from sources outside ourselves and not subject to personal control.
- *Social context*. Our social circumstances are a powerful influence on our behaviour. However, this can again be used as a means of denying responsibility for our actions. For example, some people seek to explain their behaviour as a product of their class position.

This last example is particularly significant in so far as it rests on a misunderstanding which underpins other aspects of bad faith – a confusion between *influence* and *determination*. That is, although our actions are influenced by other factors (for example, social, cultural and psychological factors), they are not determined by these factors.

However, bad faith is not simply a matter of confusing influence (pressure to behave in a certain way) with determination (our behaviour being 'caused' by external factors). Bad faith, in existentialist terms, is seen as an attempt to avoid accepting responsibility for our actions, a strategy for denying human freedom. While this may offer some degree of comfort or solace in coping with the harsh demands of human existence, it is a distorted comfort based on self-deception or, to use Sartre's phrase, it is a false salvation. As Billington (1990: 86) comments:

> I am free to reject all that I was brought up to do and believe, to turn against the mores of every community or group with which I may from time to time be identified; I am free to triumph over phobias and to conquer irrational fears. I am, in short, responsible for who I am and what I do: I cannot hold others responsible for either of these, convenient though it would sometimes be if I could. I may have been nudged, perhaps sometimes pushed, in certain directions, but in the end it is I who have chosen the way I have taken . . . To accept the determinist line seems to me an act

of surrender of one's personal sovereignty or autonomy. To do this is to begin to die.

The opposite of bad faith is *authenticity*, the full acceptance of human freedom and responsibility for our actions. It can be seen as a necessary basis for good practice:

> Authenticity, as a practice principle, is significant in two ways. First, it is a goal for workers to aim for in their own actions. In the complex, emotionally charged world of the social worker, the comfort and protection of bad faith is an inviting 'easy option' and as such is a strong temptation. However, as with all easy options, it makes a satisfactory resolution of the problems all the more difficult.
>
> Second, if clients too take the 'bad faith' escape route from their responsibilities, authenticity must be re-established before clients can take charge of their own lives and dispense with the services of a social worker. Without achieving authenticity, clients face either dependency (as they are unable to handle their own problems) or accept their problem as a long-term dimension of their existence. Social workers who rely on bad faith are in no position to help clients overcome this hurdle of self-deception and come to terms with their freedom.
>
> (Thompson 1992a: 186–7)

These examples derive from a social work context but, with only a little imagination, the transferability of the concept of authenticity to other forms of human service can be appreciated. For example, the need to take responsibility for one's own health is an important dimension of authenticity.

In addition to ontology, a central theme of existentialism is that of *phenomenology*. Phenomenology is, literally, the study of perception. It is commonly used, however, in a wider sense to refer to philosophical approaches which stress the role of meanings, values and interpretation. In this way, it is closely linked to the notion of 'hermeneutics' discussed in Chapter 3 in so far as it shares a concern with issues of subjectivity and experience. Laing (1967: 16–17) defines social phenomenology as:

> ... the science of my own and of others' experience. It is concerned with the relation between my experience of you and your experience of me. That is, with *inter-experience*. It is concerned with your behaviour and my behaviour *as I experience it*, and your and my behaviour *as you experience it*.

Phenomenology is a central part of existentialism in so far as subjective experience is seen as a fundamental reality. There is no absolute reality for us to seek out – our reality is that which we experience. This is very similar to W.I. Thomas's influential argument that, 'if a situation is defined as real, it is real in its consequences' (see Thomas and Znaniecki 1958). For example, if I assume, rightly or wrongly, that I am under threat, the fear that I experience is a real fear. The emotion becomes my experience of reality, even if that emotion were to be based on a false assumption – that is, even if the threat were not real, the fear experienced would still be very real – and my actions would be guided and informed by that experience of fear. This has a range of implications for practice, for it is to service users' subjective experiences that practitioners must respond, rather than some 'objective' reality. That is, what counts is not a particular 'event' in itself, but rather what that event *means* to the people concerned. This is not to say that objective, external factors have no part to play. Clearly they do. However, what needs to be recognized is that it is the subjective *experience* of 'objective' factors which is a major influence on human actions and values.

Phenomenology provides an important basis for understanding the importance of philosophy in the process of relating theory to practice. The term 'theory' needs to be seen in its widest sense, to incorporate phenomenological issues of meaning, perception and interpretation, as these are central to human experience. To exclude this dimension from our theory base is to subscribe to the 'technical rationality' Schön (1983, 1987) criticizes as an inadequate basis for understanding, and dealing with, the problems of the 'swampy lowlands' of practice. In this way, the neglect of the phenomenological dimension contributes

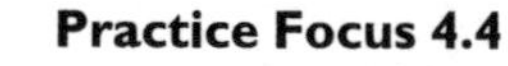

Practice Focus 4.4

Annette Davies was a 72-year-old who had lived on her own for four years since the death of her husband, Don. Dr Pearce called to see her to review her medication and was concerned about how she was managing. Consequently, the health visitor was asked to call on Mrs Davies to see whether further help was needed.

Unfortunately, however, Mrs Davies was suspicious of the doctor's motives and would therefore not let the health visitor in, as she feared that this would lead to her being 'put in a home'. The health visitor was concerned about not gaining entry and so she referred the matter to Social Services. Ironically, the arrival of the social worker to assess the situation only served to confirm Mrs Davies's fears which, by now, had become considerable. Clearly, the professionals involved in this case were going to have to deal sensitively and constructively with Mrs Davies's perceptions of the situation before being able to make progress.

to the gap between theory and practice, a topic I shall address in more detail in Chapter 5.

Lived experience

An important element within Sartre's existentialism is the concept of 'lived experience' (*le vécu*). This reflects Sartre's concern to ensure that philosophy should relate to everyday life, rather than be an abstract set of ideas with little or no connection with people's actual experience of life. Indeed, this is a central feature of existentialism, the basis of the philosophy being actual human existence – that is, *lived experience*.

This is an important issue with regard to the integration of theory and practice. For theory to have a bearing on practice, it must take account of lived experience, the subjective life-worlds of the individuals concerned. It must be able to engage with the day-to-day concerns we encounter. This does not mean that abstract concepts do not have a part to play. Clearly, these are the basic building blocks of theory. However, for theory and practice to be integrated, the concepts cannot remain at an abstract level – they have to become rooted at the concrete level (what Hall refers to as 'theorizing from the concrete' – Grossberg 1996).

It is in this respect that dialectical reason can be seen to offer a way forward in understanding the complexities of relating theory to practice. The dialectic is a means of describing and explaining movement and change – the dynamic interaction of conflicting forces. Abstract ideas and concrete reality can be seen as two such conflicting forces. It is not a question of deciding which is 'right', the abstract or the concrete, but rather understanding the interaction – and synthesis – of the two factors.

This is a fundamental premise of existentialism, that reality entails a dynamic interplay of abstract thought and concrete action. Indeed, there is a specific term to describe this – 'praxis', a fusion of thought and action. Again, this is a phenomenological perspective in so far as it presents our experience of reality not as a fixed entity or 'snapshot', but as a moving picture or, to use the technical term, a 'dialectical unfolding':

> Reality is not 'given', in the sense of being a concrete or absolute entity. It is a *construction*, a framework of perceptions and understandings based on the interplay of subjective beliefs, values and so on, and objective events, actions and circumstances.
>
> (Thompson 1992a: 183)

This has important implications for the relationship between theory and practice. Practice is not 'given', in the sense of being absolute or unchanging. Practice is a developing process, indeed a set of developing processes which interact dialectically, and so there can be no single, static theory which informs changing practice. Such a theory would very quickly lose sight of 'lived experience'.

A further aspect of lived experience is the recognition that our actions do not occur 'at random' but are geared towards particular hopes, intentions or aspirations – that is, they are future-oriented. As Mahon (1997: 7) comments:

> So human existence may, then, be seen as a project, as a constant shaping and reshaping of oneself, as a continuous choosing of objectives for oneself and a launching of oneself towards these same objectives.

Human experience, in existentialist terms, is a *process* in the sense that it is a moving, changing entity, constantly shaping and reshaping itself in line with particular plans, hopes or expectations. Lived experience, then, is not a simple event or even a series of events – the reality is far more complex than that in so far as it varies and changes in line with our evolving plans, hopes and intentions.

Existentialist practice

The discussions of existentialism as a theory base for the human services in the latter part of this chapter raise an important question: What form would an existentialist practice take? However, despite the importance of this question, a simple picture of existentialist practice is not forthcoming. This is because existentialism, by its very nature as a philosophy of freedom, rejects formula approaches with clear-cut steps to follow. That is, it would be contradictory for existentialism to dictate a prescriptive approach to practice:

> . . . existentialism is a philosophy of 'lived experience' (*le vécu*) and as such can offer the basis of a good understanding of social experience . . . However it cannot, and indeed should not, offer detailed prescriptions for practice. Existentialism is a philosophy of freedom which values personal responsibility and creativity. It would not therefore seek to tie people down to a specific range of practices and thereby predefine their practice . . . If existentialism is indeed a philosophy of lived experience, it must be true to such experience and not try to enclose it within narrow proclamations of how a particular case should be handled.
>
> (Thompson 1992a: 149)

This reflects a central theme of this book – the rejection of the simplistic notion of a direct one-to-one relationship between theory and practice. If we expect theory to provide ready-made answers to the questions practice poses, we are misunderstanding not only the nature of theory, but also of practice. Theory cannot provide simple answers which tell us 'how to do' practice. Theory can only guide and inform. Theory, practice and the relationship between them are all far too complex for there to be a clear, simple and unambiguous path for practitioners to follow. Theory provides us with the cloth from which to tailor our garment, it does not provide 'off-the-peg' solutions to practice problems.

Like other philosophies, existentialism cannot offer simple, specific solutions. However, what it can offer is a valuable way of approaching practice. In particular, it provides a basis for responding to what Schön (1992: 51) refers to as 'the indeterminate zones of practice – the situations of complexity and uncertainty'. Existentialism provides a framework for accepting uncertainty as a basic premise of human existence. While positivism stresses the quest for certainty – and conveniently sidesteps issues of uncertainty – existentialism takes uncertainty as a central concept. As Laing (1967: 47) comments:

> We must continue to struggle through our confusion, to insist on being human. Existence is a flame which constantly melts and recasts our theories. *Existential thinking offers no security*, no home for the homeless. It addresses no-one except you and me. (emphasis added)

This notion of uncertainty – of no security or guarantees – is an important one for understanding practice, particularly the 'swampy lowland where situations are confusing "messes" incapable of technical solution' (Schön 1983: 42). Dealing with uncertainty can be seen to be an important task for the practitioner. Indeed, Fish *et al.* (1989) argue that a reflective practitioner needs to have the flexibility to deal with the unique situations he or she faces – that is, the flexibility to deal with uncertainty in the absence of a formula approach which spells out exactly how the practitioner should act. This raises some important issues and so I shall return to the overlap between existentialism and reflective practice in Chapter 5. This will be in the context of exploring the notion of 'the reflective practitioner' as a means of narrowing the gap between theory and practice.

Conclusion

While the value of research was a central theme of Chapter 3, a major concern of this chapter has been the need to recognize the value of a philosophical approach. Some may see this as a contradiction, placing the 'scientific' activity of research alongside the decidedly unscientific enterprise of philosophy. However, such a view represents a gross oversimplification, a failure to recognize the complexity of the 'theory-practice problematic'. While we have seen that research has a valuable role to play, we have also seen that research has a number of limitations. We have also noted, in this chapter, that there are a number of issues which a narrow theoretical or technical approach cannot account for. This being the case, what we need to recognize is that an informed practice needs to encompass both research *and* philosophy.

This is not to deny that there is a contradiction between the two. Indeed, a tension between research and philosophy has long been recognized. However, this does not present a problem when we conceive of the two as conflicting elements within a dialectical interaction. That is, we need to understand research-based investigation and philosophical investigation as forces which interact and produce a new synthesis. They are part of a dynamic process, rather than two static entities which do not sit comfortably together.

This notion of 'dialectical reason' is perhaps one of the most important features of this chapter, as any attempt to understand theory and practice without appreciating the dialectical nature of their interaction is unlikely to get very far. In some ways, theory and practice fit neatly together but, in other ways, there is a degree of tension and conflict between them – hence the need to see them in the context of the dialectic.

Dialectical reason is the basis of the particular philosophy presented here as an appropriate and helpful basis for guiding and informing human services practice, namely the philosophy of *existentialism*. Existentialism is particularly appropriate in so far as:

- a focus on uncertainty can help practitioners to deal with the 'swampy lowlands';
- the fundamental principle of freedom and responsibility discourages dependency;
- it incorporates both the personal/individual dimension *and* the social/collective dimension;
- it provides a basis for understanding and challenging oppression;
- an understanding of ontology helps us to deal with the issues of crises and loss which human services workers so frequently encounter;
- it is premised on dialectical reason and is therefore well-equipped to deal with two of the major features of practice – change and conflict.

Of course, these benefits of an existentialist approach do not mean that existentialism should be seen as a panacea for practice. On the contrary, one of the implications of existentialism is that there can be no panacea, no easy answers, as human existence is characterized by struggle and challenge. However, what the philosophy does provide for us is an explanatory framework which helps to make sense of many of the complexities practitioners face.

This reiterates the point made at the beginning of this chapter – that philosophy is a 'subdivision' of theory (that is, a type of explanatory framework) but also *more than* theory – in the sense of being broader in its coverage of issues than the type of narrow theory associated with 'technical rationality'.

What this point illustrates is the ambiguity of the term theory. In its narrow sense, it refers to a specific, technical theory designed to account for a narrow field of study. In its broad sense, it refers to any conceptual framework designed to facilitate understanding – and this would include philosophy. From this point of view, it is clear that 'relating theory to practice' needs to be understood in terms of the broader conception of theory so that philosophical issues are also incorporated.

Food for thought

- Consider the concept of 'philosophy'.
  - What do you understand by this term?
  - How is it relevant to your work?
  - Why is it important?
- Consider the concept of 'eclecticism'.
  - What does it mean to you?
  - What are the sources of knowledge you draw on?
  - Are they incompatible in any way?
- Consider existentialism.
  - What is distinctive about this philosophical approach?
  - Are there any aspects of existentialism that you already use in your practice?
  - Are there any other aspects you could incorporate?

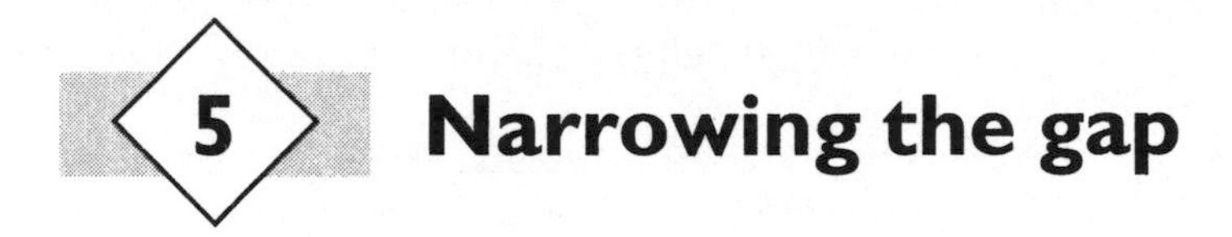

5 Narrowing the gap

Chapter overview

- Why is there a gap between theory and practice?
- What is reflective practice?
- How can it be developed?
- How can theory and practice be integrated?
- What strategies can be used?

Introduction

It is generally accepted that there is an unacceptably wide gap between theory and practice, a disjuncture between what is taught or learned and what is practised. As Buckenham and McGrath (1983: vii) put it: 'That there is a gap between the "should" of the lecture theatre and the reality of the work face is all too familiar to those intimately involved in the preparation of others for professional life'.

It is perhaps inevitable that there should be a gap between theory and practice, if only due to the fact that practice tends to change at a faster rate than theory, leaving theory in a position where it cannot catch up. There are, of course, other reasons why a separation exists between theory and practice and some of these will emerge in this chapter. However, the central issue is not whether the theory–practice gap could ever be eliminated altogether; rather, it is a matter of exploring ways in which the gap can be narrowed as far as possible, and considering how the relationship between theory and practice can be conceived and managed in a positive and constructive way.

The primary aim of this chapter is therefore twofold. First, we need to look more closely at why there is a gap between theory and practice, to consider why the two are not fully integrated. Second, we need to consider a number of strategies for 'narrowing the gap'. This entails, among other things, dispelling a number of myths about the relationship between theory and practice.

A central feature of the chapter is the concept of 'reflective practice', an approach to these issues which will act as a unifying theme. That is, the development of the notion of the 'reflective practitioner' is seen as a useful way forward in tackling these complex and thorny issues of the 'theory–practice problematic'.

Why does a gap exist?

Perhaps one of the most important reasons for the existence of a gap between theory and practice is a traditional 'division of labour' between academics and practitioners. That is, theory and practice become polarized because each is associated with a different 'camp'. Theory has come to be seen as the preserve of the academic or educator, and practice is seen as being within the domain of the practitioner. To what extent the two groups can work effectively together is an interesting and important question.

Both camps can become entrenched in their respective positions. From an academic point of view, this happens when elitism is allowed to come to the fore. This is when theory development is seen as superior to, or more important than, practice development, thereby creating barriers, suspicion and mistrust. In this way, elitism maintains a considerable distance between theory and practice.

From a practice point of view, the position can become entrenched as a result of anti-intellectualism. This involves a rejection of theoretical or intellectual matters on the grounds that they are deemed to be irrelevant to practice – out of touch with reality. Educators are seen to inhabit 'ivory towers' where they have little insight into the world of practice, and where they are cushioned from the harsh realities of the demands of practice.

Anti-intellectualism can take one of two forms – strong or weak. The weak form involves the 'I prefer to stick to practice' attitude, which presents theory as an irrelevance of little or no concern to practitioners. This approach is characterized by a tendency to ignore the existence of theory and to practise in an uncritical, routine way. The strong form, by contrast, extends beyond this and is more aggressive in its rejection of theory. This approach is characterized by not simply ignoring theory, but by actively rejecting it, for example through ridicule.

Of course, part of the attraction of anti-intellectualism is that it offers a degree of protection from criticism. Any critique of a practitioner's work which goes beyond simple, day-to-day concepts can be dismissed or disregarded as 'theory' and therefore seen as invalid on the grounds that it is out of touch with reality – the narrowly circumscribed simplistic 'reality' of those practitioners who see the world of ideas as separate from the world of practice. In this way, anti-intellectualism can be seen as a form of bad faith.

However, the polarization of theory and practice is not simply a matter of attitudes. There are also wider issues to consider. In particular, we need to recognize organizational pressures which can have the effect of driving theory and practice apart. For example, workload demands on practitioners can prevent them from finding the 'thinking time' necessary for reflecting on their practice and adopting a more informed approach. Similarly, academic staff may be under pressure to produce research and develop theory, perhaps at the expense of drawing out the practice implications of existing knowledge and research. Such constraints are not absolute barriers to the integration of theory and practice for, as we shall see below, steps can be taken to minimize their impact. Their significance should none the less be noted.

A further reason for the existence of a gap between theory and practice is one that has already been commented on in Chapter 2, namely the mystique that has come to be associated with theory. This mystique is partly explained by reference to the elitism mentioned above, the tendency to see theory as superior to practice.

Such a mystique has the effect of discouraging practitioners from engaging with theory issues, as such matters are seen as being 'above

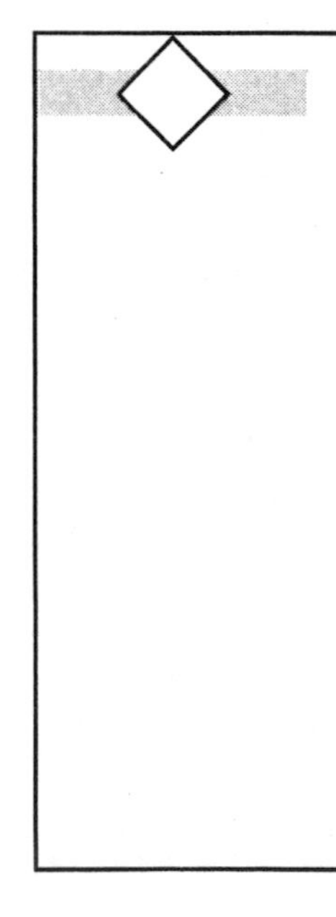

Practice Focus 5.1

Sian had enjoyed the first year of her course, particularly her practical experience. She had also learned a great deal from her studies but felt rather distanced from some of the academic content of the course – she was in awe of 'intellectuals'. In effect, she was a victim of the 'mystique' of theory.

However, shortly after the beginning of the second year of the course, she attended a lecture given by a guest speaker who happened to be the author of one of the textbooks used on the course. Sian was amazed to find how 'ordinary' the author turned out to be, quite down-to-earth and easy to relate to, quite unlike her image of the author of a theoretical book. After the lecture, Sian commented on this to some of her fellow students and found that most of them felt the same way. The discussion that followed from this helped her to feel more confident about theory. This was to be her first step towards overcoming the mystique of theory.

their heads'. In this way, the mystique of theory can instigate a vicious circle. The mystique of theory discourages the use of theory which, in turn, reinforces that mystique, and the separation which it engenders.

The crux of this situation is that seeing theory as 'beyond the grasp' of practitioners creates a self-fulfilling prophecy – the presumed superiority of theory creates a distance between theory and practice. It places theory on a pedestal and thus perpetuates the mystique. And yet this mystique, ironically, is based on a fallacy. It makes no sense to describe theory as superior to practice, as this fails to recognize the close inter-dependence of the two. As Susser (1968: v) comments: 'to practice without theory is to sail an uncharted sea; theory without practice is not to set sail at all' (cited in Hardiker and Barker 1991: 87).

In addition to the problem of the mystique of theory, the popularity of eclecticism can also be seen as a barrier to the integration of theory and practice. As was noted in Chapter 4, a tendency to mix elements of theory in an uncritical and unplanned way only pays lip service to the notion of relating theory to practice. By 'going through the motions' in this way, a semblance of integration is produced, whereas in reality all that is achieved is a hotch-potch. The goal of an informed practice is therefore not achieved by eclecticism. Indeed, we can even go so far as to say that achieving such a goal is hindered by eclecticism in so far as it discourages practitioners from looking more closely and critically at the ideas underpinning their practice. It is therefore important that we develop alternatives to eclecticism, a point to which I shall return below.

Developing reflective practice

The concept of 'reflective practice' has become relatively well-established in nurse education but has had a lower level of influence in other forms of human service education. Its primary value is in the way in which it unites theory and practice within the same framework, without presenting either as being in any way superior to the other. It is therefore worth exploring further the notion of reflective practice so that its role in integrating theory and practice can be more fully understood and appreciated.

Gould (1996: 1) comments on the value of reflective practice:

> There is considerable empirical evidence, based on research into a variety of occupations, suggesting that expertise does not derive from the application of rules or procedures applied deductively from positivist research. Instead, it is argued that practice wisdom rests upon highly developed intuition which may be difficult to articulate but can be demonstrated through practice. On the basis of this reconstructed epistemology of practice, reflective learning

> offers an approach to education which operates through an understanding of professional knowledge as primarily developed through practice and the systematic analysis of experience.

The development of reflective practice owes much to the work of Donald Schön (1983, 1987, 1992). His writings have had a major impact on our understanding of the relationship between theory and practice. He introduced a number of key concepts which have proved very influential. Of particular value is the notion of 'reflection-in-action'. Schön describes practice in terms of what he calls a 'reflective conversation with the situation'. This offers a significantly different perspective on the use of theory, a perspective which goes beyond the traditional polarization of theory and practice brought about by an emphasis on 'technical rationality':

> According to the model of Technical Rationality, there is an objectively knowable world, independent of the practitioner's values and views. In order to gain technical knowledge of it, the practitioner must maintain a clear boundary between himself and his object of inquiry . . . In a practitioner's reflective conversation with a situation that he treats as unique and uncertain, he functions as an agent/experient. Through his transaction with the situation, he shapes it and makes himself a part of it. Hence, the sense he makes of the situation must include his own contribution to it. Yet he recognizes that the situation, having a life of its own distinct from his intentions, may foil his projects and reveal new meanings.
>
> (Schön 1983: 163)

This is an important passage, as it highlights a number of important aspects of reflective practice:

- Conventional approaches which rely on technical rationality offer an inadequate basis for guiding and informing professional practice.
- Using theory in practice involves a 'reflective conversation with the situation'. This implies a *phenomenological* approach which emphasizes the active interpretation of events. This shows the inappropriateness of approaches which seek a simple formula for applying theory to practice.
- Uncertainty is a key issue in professional practice (Schön's 'swampy lowlands') and so the ability to handle uncertainty is an important skill for practitioners to develop.
- Practitioners become 'part of the situation' when they engage in their professional duties. Attempts to remain 'objective' are therefore unrealistic. What needs to be addressed is the interplay of subjective and objective factors (as discussed in Chapter 4).
- Our projects can be 'foiled' by aspects of the situation which work

against what we are trying to achieve. In this respect, no theory can offer guarantees of success.

These five pointers help to paint a picture of reflective practice as a very different enterprise from the simplistic common sense idea of fitting the square peg of theory into the round hole of practice. Theory cannot be seen as an entity that can simply be taken 'off the shelf' and applied to practice in a mechanistic way. It is better conceived of as an interactive process through which concepts and frameworks are 'made to measure' by the skilful work of the reflective practitioner. As Vince (1996: 1) puts it, practitioners need: 'to continually theorise their practice and practise their theory'. In this way, human services practice, although based on 'science', is also very much a craft – a highly skilled activity that goes beyond the direct application of technical skills..

The above five pointers also paint another picture – one in which the parallels between reflective practice and existentialism can be identified. Like reflective practice, existentialism:

- goes beyond technical rationality;
- has a basis in phenomenology;
- acknowledges the significance of uncertainty;
- emphasizes the interplay of subjective and objective factors; and
- recognizes that there can be no guarantees.

A central premise of existentialism is that human action needs to be understood in terms of 'the person in situation'. This relates to the dialectical interaction of the individual's *subjective* experience (the person) and the *objective* context in which it occurs (the situation). This is very similar to the basis of reflective practice: the struggle to make sense of (and deal with) the complex interaction of factors within the 'indeterminate zones of practice – the situations of

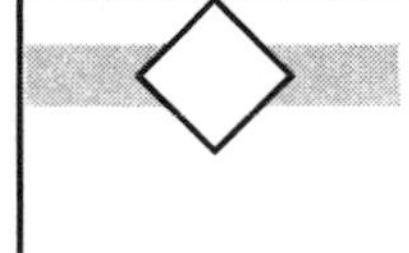

Practice Focus 5.2

Ian was the manager of a social education centre for people with learning difficulties. He was pleased to be offered the chance to study for a certificate in management studies as he was keen to improve his skills. However, he was disappointed by the outcome as he could not see simple and direct links between the knowledge he was acquiring and the demands of his job.

Ian had fallen foul of the 'osmosis' approach to learning. He had assumed that, simply by absorbing knowledge, his practice skills as a manager would improve. He had not realized that learning has to be tailored to fit the circumstances – a craft as well as a science.

complexity and uncertainty, the unique cases that require artistry, the elusive task of problem-setting' (Schön 1992: 51). Both existentialism and reflective practice go beyond a mechanistic view of applying theory to practice and recognize the subtle intricacies involved in the fusion of thought and action.

The analogy used above is an important one, namely the conception of theory–practice integration as 'tailor-made', rather than 'off the peg'. Theoretical approaches are often rejected by some students and practitioners because they do not match up closely with the practice situations they encounter – that is, theory does not 'fit' practice. The problem inherent in this situation is that it assumes that theory should relate directly and unambiguously to practice with little need to make adjustments to either theory or practice.

This attitude towards theory–practice integration is unhelpful in so far as it underestimates the complexities of relating theory to practice. Evans (1990: 30) gives us a picture of how complex the process of applying theory to practice is:

> 'Application' has a number of different meanings. It can mean taking a theory and putting it into practice. I have known a number of students who came on placements fired with ideas and seeking to impose them on people with unfortunately ill-matched social problems. A second meaning is that commonly applied in case studies: a piece of practice is retrospectively analysed and different theoretical labels are applied to it.
>
> A more subtle understanding of 'applying' however, is the recognition of certain factors within a practice situation which certain knowledge or theory might benefit. The knowledge or theory then needs to be shaped by a process of concretisation . . . to the specific practice context before it can be of benefit.

The term 'concretisation' is a key word here. Theory has to be made concrete, brought down to earth as it were. For example, behavioural therapy can offer a clear framework for practice but has to be adapted to suit the specific circumstances of the practice situation – it cannot be applied in a blanket fashion to all situations.

Shaping the theory for the practice context is a key part of the process and illustrates well the idea of theory having to be tailor-made for practice, rather than simply tagged-on to practice in an uncritical way. As Evans goes on to suggest, this is no simple or straightforward matter. It is therefore important that we consider some strategies for developing reflective practice in particular, and integrating theory and practice in general. However, before undertaking this task, it is worth devoting some time to identifying one of the key weaknesses of reflective practice as it is currently understood.

Beyond reflection

The literature relating to reflective practice is part of what could broadly be described as an adult education paradigm. As such, it is concerned mainly with the interaction between the individual learner and his or her learning environment. While this is quite apt as far as it goes, it can be argued that it does not go far enough. That is, reflective practice is premised on individualism and does not take account of wider social and political factors or of the organizational context in which practice takes place.

The work of Schön, for example, makes little or no reference to the sociopolitical factors which can have a major impact on the context in which learning and practice take place. Such factors include the significance of issues of gender, race, culture, disability and so on. As was noted in Chapter 1, such matters are important dimensions of human action and interaction, and to neglect these is to run the risk of (unwittingly) perpetrating or reinforcing discrimination and oppression. In this regard, Vince (1996: 33) makes apt comment:

> One of the most fundamental propositions informing experiential learning is the notion that the review and development of individual experience forms the basic resource for learning (Smith, 1980). It often seems that such learning, because it focuses on the individual, is somehow detached from the social and political context of experience. Both individual and collective experience are invariable products of a social system, and in turn contribute to the capacity of that system to resist change. In other words, our experience is both conditioned by, and an exercise of, power (Roberts, 1996).

However, this is not an intrinsic fault which cannot be rectified. The neglect of broader issues can be seen as an area for development, rather than a fatal flaw which stands in the way of progress. Indeed, the beginnings of such a development are already apparent. For example, Mezirow (1981) introduces the concept of 'perspective transformation', a process which can be seen to act as a bridge between reflective practice and anti-discriminatory practice. Perspective transformation is a term used to refer to:

> . . . the emancipatory process of *becoming critically aware of how and why the structure of psycho-cultural assumptions has come to constrain the way we see ourselves and our relationships, reconstituting this structure to permit a more inclusive and discriminating integration of experience and acting upon these new understandings.*
>
> (Mezirow 1981: 6)

Or, to put it more simply, perspective transformation is the process by which we can set ourselves free from hidebound patterns of thought and action – the types of pattern which derive from the cultural and social influences to which we are constantly exposed. As Mezirow (1981: 6–7) goes on to say: 'It is the learning process by which adults come to recognize their culturally induced dependency roles and relationships and the reasons for them and take action to overcome them'.

It is in this way that perspective transformation can be seen as an important linkage between reflective practice and anti-discriminatory practice. It is relevant to reflective practice in so far as perspective transformation can be the outcome of reflection. By reflecting on practice, assumptions and established 'mind-sets' can be identified, challenged and overcome. Similarly, perspective transformation has a significant bearing on anti-discriminatory practice.

Developing forms of practice which are sensitive to discrimination and oppression involves challenging common-sense assumptions which lead to inequality and disadvantage, for example racial or gender stereotypes. This involves 'unlearning' patterns of socialization, casting off dominant attitudes and values which reinforce discriminatory and oppressive ideologies such as racism, sexism and so on. This unlearning is, therefore, a form of perspective transformation – it involves developing our own perspective, rather than simply accepting uncritically dominant ideas and values. It is in this sense that perspective transformation is an 'emancipatory process':

> The process involves what Freire calls 'problem-posing', making problematic our taken-for-granted social roles and expectations and the habitual ways we act and feel in carrying them out. The resulting transformation in perspective or personal paradigm is what Freire refers to as 'conscientization' and Habermas as emancipatory action.
>
> (Mezirow 1981: 7)

Perspective transformation is therefore a helpful concept in developing a practice which is both reflective and anti-discriminatory. What it also succeeds in doing is to develop a clearer understanding of the broader social and political context. Both theory and practice exist within a framework of values, power, social forces and social institutions. Relating theory to practice therefore needs to be seen within a sociopolitical context. To ignore this context is therefore to adopt a narrow and blinkered view which is likely to stand in the way of further progress. This is a point to which I shall return in Chapter 6.

Similarly, we can see that the significance of the organizational context in which theory and practice are integrated is not generally given the attention it deserves. It is for this reason that Chapter 7 includes a consideration of organizational factors.

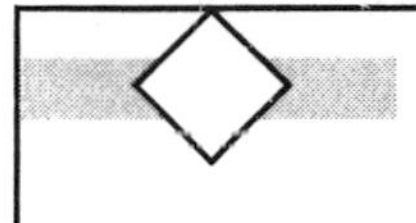

Practice Focus 5.3

Bill was keen to do well on his social work course and he was particularly keen to address issues of social deprivation and racism, as he had become very aware of these problems during his upbringing. However, what he was not particularly aware of were problems of sexism. The course's commitment to developing anti-sexist practice was something he had not bargained for.

At first, he was very resistant to the ideas and felt that the significance of sexism in social work was being overstated. However, as the course progressed, he gradually realized just how important a role gender played in social problems and the provision of services. What really brought the point home to him was a workshop on sexual abuse in which he was shocked to realize the significance of the association between power and male sexuality in relation to sexual abuse. It was only now that the danger of taking gender expectations for granted struck him as being of such importance.

Following this he was far more attuned to gender issues and he went from strength to strength in developing anti-sexist practice. He found it difficult to believe that he had previously accepted gender roles and expectations so uncritically. That is, he was only just beginning to adjust to the 'perspective transformation' he had undergone.

Integrating theory and practice

One of the recurring themes of this book is that relating theory to practice is not a simple, mechanistic process. It is better understood as a more complex and subtle fusion of thoughts, feelings, actions and values. As we have seen, theory and practice are often integrated with little or no conscious thought involved in the process, as the concept of the 'fallacy of theoryless practice' implies.

In this way, theory – or some aspects of theory at least – becomes more or less automatically fused with practice, as captured by Schön's (1983) phrase 'knowledge-in-action'. The knowledge is somehow 'in' the action. This being the case, the question could be posed: If theory and practice tend to be fused spontaneously, why do we need to worry about relating theory to practice? The answer to this is contained, partly at least, in the comments of Preston-Shoot and Agass (1990: 8):

> No one can be atheoretical. Values, culture, gender, socialisation and professional training all shape our theories and belief systems which we take into life and work which must, therefore, be owned and critically appraised. Otherwise, social workers may

leave some areas unexplored and become boxed in by their own bias.

Although theory and practice do become fused, we need to take control of this process as far as possible so that we can:

- be conscious of the potential for bias and discrimination;
- make the best and most constructive use of the knowledge available;
- maximize opportunities for learning (and, indirectly, job satisfaction);
- challenge and develop the knowledge base;
- avoid the mistakes of the past.

This final point is particularly significant for, as Douglas (1986: 11) comments: 'Traditional approaches perpetuate mistakes as well as good practice'.

Theory and practice do become integrated, but this is often in an uncritical, haphazard and uncoordinated way. There is, therefore, considerable benefit in making this integration more deliberate and explicit so that its benefits can be fully exploited and its pitfalls avoided. That is, it is not simply a question of achieving the integration of theory and practice – this occurs anyway – but, rather, achieving the *optimal* integration of the two. As Boud and Walker (1990: 66) comment:

> In any experience there may be reflective activity occurring in which what the learner perceives is processed and becomes the basis of new knowledge and further action. Information is associated with previous knowledge, is integrated with it, and may then be tested in the event. *Reflection is a normal on-going process which can, if desired, be made more explicit and more ordered.* (emphasis added)

In order to assist in this process of making the fusion of thought and action 'more explicit and more ordered', a number of strategies for integrating theory and practice can be identified. It is to these that we now turn.

Strategies for integration

Fifteen strategies in total are presented here. These are offered as a means of facilitating the optimal integration of theory and practice. However, this list is neither comprehensive nor definitive, but can take us some significant way forward in addressing these issues. Of course, it would run counter to the spirit of reflective practice if I, as a theorist, were to propose a comprehensive set of step-by-step guidelines for developing reflective practice. What is presented here is intended as a stimulus to the development of reflective practice, rather than a blueprint for doing so. It is to be hoped that the examples given here will encourage readers – both individually and collectively – to consider, develop and use strategies of their own.

Using cycles of learning

In Chapter 1, Kolb's learning cycle was presented as a model for understanding adult learning. Learning arises as a result of the four-stage process of: concrete experience; reflective observation; abstract conceptualization; and active experimentation. This is a model which can also be used to describe, and facilitate, the integration of theory and practice.

Theory and practice are both a part of a wider cycle of learning. The cycle begins with concrete experience, which is then reflected upon and related to previous learning and experience, before being tried out again in practice. This represents a process in which theory and practice interact and become merged. Morrison (1993: 45) quotes the Further Education Unit (1988) in this regard:

> It is not sufficient to have an experience to learn. Without reflecting on the experience it may be lost or misunderstood. It is from feelings and thoughts emerging from this reflection that generalisations and concepts can be generated. It is from generalisations that we become better able to tackle new situations.
>
> Similarly, if we want behaviour to change by learning, developing new concepts alone will not be effective. The learning must be tested out in new situations through active experimentation. This is how we link theory and action. If this is not done, we may get it 'right' but without knowing why. Then we will not be able to repeat it in a similar situation.

What this emphasizes is that learning and relating theory to practice are both part of an active, cyclical process. An important strategy, therefore, for integrating theory and practice is to engage with this process, to enter fully and explicitly into the cycle of learning from experience, as described by Kolb and his colleagues (Morrison 1993, offers useful guidelines in this respect).

Going beyond practice wisdom

Practice is often seen as an art or craft, as distinct from the 'science' of theory. There is a danger, however, in taking this analogy too far. Just as theory can become mystified, so too can the 'art' of practice. This is a dangerous development where it occurs, as such a view acts as a barrier to the constructive use of theory – it devalues theory and formal knowledge. As Schön (1983: 276) comments:

> According to conventional wisdom, thinking interferes with doing in two ways. First, artistry being indescribable, reflection on action is doomed to failure, and second, reflection-in-action paralyzes action. Both arguments are largely, though not entirely, mistaken. They owe their plausibility to the persistence of misleading views about the relation of thought to action.

An over-reliance on practice wisdom is therefore both misleading and unhelpful. It presents one element within a dialectical interaction as if it were largely unconnected with the other. It presents a distorted and simplistic view of what is a complex and subtle process.

As we have noted, informal, uncodified theory has an important part to play in guiding and informing practice. Relating theory to practice does not simply mean trying to make use of 'textbook' theory. It involves drawing on a range of sources – some formal, some informal – and using these constructively where appropriate. That is, the theory base of practice is an extensive one and so its use needs to be 'tailor-made', rather than 'off the peg'. Becoming too dependent on practice wisdom will therefore tend to produce too much of a standard 'off-the-peg' approach, as it fails to recognize the value and significance of the process of 'tailoring'.

A major implication of this argument is that conscious efforts need to be made to go beyond practice wisdom. Without such efforts, the temptation to 'rest on our laurels' is likely to prove too strong for us to resist (see also Thompson 1996, Chapter 20).

Going beyond theoryless practice

As we have seen, the question of practice without theory does not arise, as practice is inevitably imbued with ideas, values and assumptions. The question therefore is not *whether* to use theory, but rather *how* to use theory to best effect. In this respect, the false belief in a theoryless practice has much in common with an over-reliance on practice wisdom in so far as both undervalue the use of theory in a direct and explicit way as a means of guiding and enhancing practice.

By failing to recognize the fallacy of theoryless practice, we fail to take account of the assumptions underpinning our practice. As Roberts (1990: 35) comments:

> In the case of a person who believes his behaviour is not connected to any theory, it can be assumed, argues Johnson (1981), that the action is connected to a theory of some kind, but this theory remains unacknowledged by the person because he or she may be unaware of the assumptions being made.

The simplest way to understand this situation is to divide practitioners into two groups: those who recognize the influence of theoretical knowledge on practice and seek to benefit from it; and those who ignore or reject the role of theory and thereby run the risk of basing their practice on false assumptions. Clearly, the potential for dangerous practice is significantly higher for the second group. As Lecomte (1975: 209) argues: 'It is the theory used by a practitioner without knowing he is using it that is dangerous to practitioners and their clients' (quoted in Roberts 1990: 35).

It is therefore important that we sensitize ourselves to the fallacy of theoryless practice so that we do not become complacent about the dangers of neglecting the influence of ideas, values and assumptions on our actions. A simple, but none the less essential strategy, therefore, is to ensure that we do not lose sight of the theoretical foundations of our practice, that we do not fall into the trap of 'overlearning'.

Going beyond common sense

In Chapter 1, the dangers of relying on common sense were commented on, particularly in relation to anti-discriminatory practice. The point about common sense, however, is that it is, by its very nature, deeply ingrained. 'Common sense' is, to a large extent, a shorthand for dominant cultural values, the ideology – or sets of ideologies – into which we are socialized from an early age.

This is not to say that common sense is necessarily 'wrong' or inappropriate. Indeed, much of our so-called common-sense knowledge derives from sociological research (Giddens 1993b) and has therefore been subjected to some degree of rigorous testing. But, the significant point to note is that common-sense beliefs – whether based in fact or ideology – are *unquestioned* beliefs. They are based on assumption, rather than assessment and analysis.

This is another aspect of the ideological nature of common sense – the tendency for statements like 'It's common sense . . .' to be used as a means of deterring critical reflection. 'Common sense' is used as a tactic for closing debates, rather than opening them. To argue that a particular point of view is 'just common sense' is a powerful way of discouraging people from challenging that point of view. Many people will not be prepared to risk being seen to go against common sense. Common sense is therefore ideological in two senses: much of the content of common-sense beliefs derives from dominant ideological values and assumptions; and common sense protects dominant ideological perspectives by deterring critical thinking. A reliance on common sense can therefore act as a stumbling block to the optimal integration of theory and practice. Common sense therefore raises questions rather than provides answers. An important strategy, therefore, is to be wary of common sense and to maintain a critical perspective, one based on thought rather than thoughtless assumption.

Developing research-minded practice

At the end of Chapter 3, I presented Everitt and co-workers' (1992) concept of 'research-minded practice' as a helpful basis for integrating theory and practice. I described it as a term which captures both elements of best practice – an effective combination of intellectual inquiry and pragmatic application.

Research-minded practice involves recognizing the parallel between research activity and human services practice. Schön (1983: 147) comments on the similarities between research and professional practice:

> If a carpenter asks himself, What makes this structure stable? and begins to experiment to find out – trying now one device, now another – he is basically in the same business as the research scientist. He puts forward hypotheses and, within the limits of the constraining features of the practice context, tries to discriminate among them – taking as disconfirmation of a hypothesis the failure to get the consequences predicted from it. The logic of this experimental inference is the same as the researcher's.

For research to be accepted as valid, it has to have some degree of rigour and discipline, but also has to draw on a measure of creativity

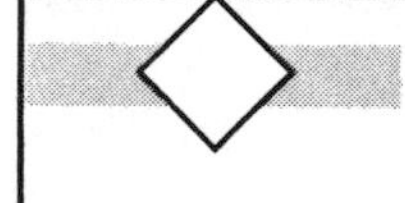

Practice Focus 5.4

Denise was an experienced health visitor who had recently been given special responsibility for child protection. She had a great deal of experience of this type of work but was anxious about her new responsibilities. Consequently, she took the opportunity to seek guidance from a number of experienced child protection professionals as part of her induction programme.

She sought advice on a number of issues but two themes kept recurring. First, she noticed that there was an emphasis on the need to follow the child protection procedures, to be rigorous and thorough in ensuring that the necessary safeguards were put in place. Second, she noted the emphasis on the need to be creative and imaginative, to develop an extensive repertoire of methods of working with children and their families in difficult and distressing circumstances. The fundamental lesson she learned from this process, then, was the need to find the optimal balance between rigour and creativity.

and imaginative investigation. Human services practice can also benefit from this successful blend of rigour and creativity. Research-minded practice aims to achieve this balance.

Research and practice, however, are also very different in some respects. For example, the focus of research is on understanding, whereas for practice the focus is on producing change. None the less, it remains the case that research and practice have much to benefit from each other. In this respect, research-minded practice seeks to achieve the best of both worlds.

A key aspect of developing research-minded practice is to adopt a *participative* approach, one based on partnership, rather than paternalism:

> Practice can be improved, too, by being imbued with clarity of thought, critical analysis and informed choice of approach. Both empowering practice and empowering research depend on being participatory, encouraging participants to 'own' the outcome by setting the goals and sharing in decisions about the most desirable process to be followed.
>
> (Everitt *et al.* 1992: 50)

A participative approach therefore contributes to demystifying both research and practice, and thereby brings the two closer together.

Going beyond elitism and anti-intellectualism

These two factors, elitism and anti-intellectualism, have already been noted as significant barriers to the integration of theory and practice. Elitism results from, and contributes to, a sense of intellectual snobbery – a belief that the world of ideas is superior to, or more important than, the world of practice. Conversely, anti-intellectualism attaches little or no significance or value to the role of theory. Theoretical ideas are seen as an irrelevance, or even as a barrier to effective practice.

In order to reduce the possibility of elitism and anti-intellectualism hindering the integration of theory and practice, both academics and practitioners have a part to play – a shared responsibility for breaking down barriers. Academics and educators have a duty to eschew elitism and to make theory and formal knowledge accessible to practitioners and applicable to practice. Rafferty (1992: 509) argues that:

> . . . unless theory can be applied to enhance practice it has no meaning in the real world . . . If students are not to be caught between unrealistic expectations on the part of educationalists and the real world of practice, then teachers must teach realistically and apply the curriculum accordingly. This is not to say that there should be any compromise of standards, but if teaching is esoteric and unrealistic, students will have false

> expectations and may be frustrated and confused when they encounter the clinical environment.

This passage captures well the need for theory and education to be practice-focused. However, it is significant to note that the passage also reveals a tendency towards anti-intellectualism. There are two references to the world of practice as the 'real' world, as if theory and research were not part of this 'real' world.

This illustrates the difficult balance which needs to be found, a balance which avoids the destructive extremes of elitism and anti-intellectualism. Finding the means to achieve this balance can therefore be seen as an important strategy for bringing theory and practice together.

Using the critical incident technique

As we have noted, reflective practice represents a successful blend of theory and practice. A useful way to promote reflective practice is the 'critical incident technique'. This is a method which can be used on training courses, in team or staff meetings, or in discussions within the context of a supervisory relationship.

Wright (1989: 34) defines a critical incident as:

> ... any situation faced by emergency and critical care personnel that causes them to experience unusually strong emotional reactions. These feelings have the potential to interfere with their ability to function either at the time, or later.

However, other writers tend to use a broader definition. For example, Smith and Russell (1991: 286) refers to Clamp's (1980) definition of critical incidents as 'snapshot views of the daily work of the nurse'. For present purposes, I shall use the term in the sense of any incident which makes a particular impact or impression on the staff concerned.

A simple way of using the critical incident technique involves asking the student/practitioner to identify a particular critical incident, to reflect upon it and to address the following three questions (based on Smith and Russell 1993):

1. What happened in this incident?
2. How would you account for this?
3. What other conceptual frameworks could help us understand this incident?

This simple but effective framework provides an excellent basis for discussion and exploration of the linkages between theory and practice in a way which enhances practice and brings theory to life. It is a technique which can be used on a one-to-one basis or as part of a group exercise.

An important point to note, however, in using this technique is that it can often generate strong emotions. Incidents encountered can have a powerful emotional impact and the analysis of the incident can rekindle intense and painful feelings. This has two sets of implications:

1. Facilitators need to be ready and able to work constructively with such feelings as and when they arise, for example by creating a safe environment.
2. It needs to be remembered that theory has a role to play in dealing with the emotional dimension of human services practice. We need to be wary of the false assumption that theory is 'rational', and therefore incompatible with the 'irrational' world of feelings.

The use of the critical incident technique therefore represents an important and potentially very effective strategy for integrating theory and practice.

Developing a group approach

A further possible technique for narrowing the gap between theory and practice is the development of learning sets. A learning set is an extension of the notion of 'quality circle' which derives from management theory:

> Quality circles (QC), or quality control circles, comprise groups of workers and supervisors in a single area or department in an organization, which meet regularly to study ways of improving production quality, and to monitor progress towards such goals. Developed originally in Japan, QC are now widespread in most industries in the West. They provide, in effect, an organizational device depending upon participation and motivation to help achieve quality during manufacture.
>
> (in Kempner 1987: 430)

By setting up a group of people to take responsibility for one or more aspects of quality, staff can be helped to develop a sense of involvement, ownership and empowerment. Members of a quality circle can not only contribute to improving quality but also learn a great deal in the process.

This can then be taken a step further in the form of a 'learning set'. This term describes a group set up specifically to promote learning and develop a better understanding of a particular issue or set of issues – a quality circle geared specifically towards the quality of learning and staff development in an organization or part of an organization. An example of this would be a group of staff with responsibility for students engaged in work-based training deciding to hold a series of regular meetings to share experiences and maximize their opportunities for learning. Such a group would constitute a learning set and could provide an excellent basis for developing reflective practice, and thereby linking theory and practice. A group approach also provides opportunities for mutual support and the critical exploration of ideas in a safe, supportive environment where the theory–practice relationship can be explored more fully and effectively. Consequently, this approach can be seen to have much to commend it in terms of facilitating the integration of theory and practice. Seeking opportunities to develop learning sets, wherever possible and appropriate, therefore amounts to a further important basic strategy for bringing together theory and practice in an effective and coherent way. Its particular strength is that it promotes a sense of ownership and shared responsibility – it discourages the tendency to cut off practice from its theoretical roots.

Promoting continuous professional development

Continuous professional development (or CPD as it has become known) is a concept which has become increasingly well-established in recent years in the literature relating to training and staff development. It refers to the recognition of the need for ongoing opportunities for learning and development beyond the point of initial qualification. It is an approach which seeks to counter the not uncommon tendency to regard achieving a professional qualification as the end of a process of learning, rather than the entry point into a new phase of learning.

CPD can be seen to comprise three main elements:

1. *In-service training*: involvement in training courses is an important part of forming and strengthening links between ideas and actions.
2. *Supervision*: the effective use of line management structures can be a major source of learning and professional development. It offers scope for evaluating practice and exploring a range of possible interventions (Morrison 1993).
3. *Appraisal*: this is often viewed in negative terms, as a means of 'checking-up' on staff. However, where it is used constructively and effectively, it helps workers maintain a clear focus on what they are trying to achieve and how they intend to achieve it.

These three elements are major building blocks of continuous professional development. They contribute to maintaining motivation and commitment, and thereby increase opportunities for job satisfaction.

CPD, though, is not only a significant source of motivation, it is also an important vehicle for the optimal integration of theory and practice. It provides an excellent context for such integration by encouraging staff to continue to think about their practice and continually seek out new and better ways of working. In short, it provides fertile soil for the development of reflective practice.

Without an emphasis on CPD, there is a danger that staff will practise in a routine, uncritical way and lose sight of the values and knowledge base that underpin practice. This can lead to complacency, a lack of alertness and sensitivity, and ultimately perhaps, burnout (Thompson *et al.* 1994a).

The strategy to be developed here, therefore, is one of establishing a commitment to continuous professional development, an attitude which sees learning as an essential component of good practice.

Developing interprofessional learning

Although the knowledge, skills and values underpinning practice have much in common across the different human services fields, it is surprising that there is relatively little interprofessional education and training. Opportunities for shared learning are in plentiful supply when we consider that each professional field has its own perspectives and insights to bring to common areas of concern (communication, for example). The possibilities for generating reflective learning opportunities through interprofessional education and training can be seen as a largely unexplored area.

An important postmodernist concept is that of 'dedifferentiation'. This refers to the need to break down arbitrary and unhelpful barriers between academic disciplines. For example, much social psychology overlaps considerably with some forms of microsociology, and yet the boundaries between the two disciplines generally remain intact, often acting as barriers to further theory development. The same argument could also be applied to professional fields, with considerable scope for the transfer of learning from one discipline to another (Thompson and Bates 1996).

This can also be seen from the literature available. Consider, for example, two important books on reflective practice: Palmer *et al.* (1994) and Gould and Taylor (1996). The former is entitled *Reflective Practice in Nursing*, while the latter is called *Reflective Learning for Social Work*. While the two books are very different in a number of ways, they also have much in common. Indeed, social workers could learn much from reading the nursing text and nurses could benefit from what is on offer in the social work book. While not wishing to underplay the significant differences between the two professional groups, the notion of 'dedifferentiation' could clearly be of benefit here, not only to social workers and nurses, but also to the other professional groups within the human services.

Using mentoring

The notion of 'mentoring' has been around for a long time, mainly as an informal process that occurs between experienced 'old hands' and relative newcomers. However, it is increasingly being used in a more formal sense, particularly in relation to postqualifying or postregistration education and training. The mentor's role is not so much that of a direct teacher (although elements of direct teaching may feature) as that of a facilitator of learning – someone who asks the type of questions that stimulate a reflective analysis of practice so that the benefits of experiential learning can be maximized.

The use of practice teachers, student supervisors, clinical teachers and so on has a long history in the human services, and clearly such roles have contributed significantly to professional development. However, such roles are generally associated with staff at the beginning of their careers or those seeking to transfer from unqualified to qualified status. The notion of mentoring goes far beyond this, being applicable to all staff at all stages in their career. Access to an experienced and supportive colleague who is skilled in facilitating learning is something that all staff can benefit from as part of a commitment to reflective practice in particular and continuous professional development in general. Indeed, if the notion of continuous professional development is to be taken seriously, then the question of mentoring for *all* staff certainly comes onto the agenda.

It could be argued that such mentoring already occurs for many people through supervision and appraisal systems. While it is certainly true that line management supervision *can* involve an important mentoring role, it is clearly not the case that all supervision incorporates an element of mentoring. Conversely, excellent mentoring relationships can exist outside of formal reporting structures or line management systems. Mentoring can therefore overlap with supervision but cannot be equated with it.

Problematizing

This is a term used to refer to the process of making the ordinary extraordinary. That is, many opportunities for learning and improving practice can be masked beneath the veneer of everyday routines and standard practices – problematizing involves uncovering these opportunities. As Griseri (1998: 17) comments:

> Ellen Langer talks of the negative effects of taking things for granted, which she calls 'mindlessness'. In contrast, she points out how creativity and greater understanding can often be stimulated by focusing on what one has always accepted and regarding it as no longer certain.

It is inevitable that we will rely, up to a point on routines and ways of operating that require the minimum of thought. For many tasks we need to have this mindlessness to be able to get through without overloading ourselves or falling into the trap of 'paralysis by analysis'. The technique of problematizing therefore involves identifying one or more such aspects of our work and then questioning it so that we:

- create opportunities for seeing the situation from a different, perhaps broader perspective;
- avoid complacency and an over-reliance on routines;
- facilitate a reflective approach.

It is interesting to note that this process of problematizing often happens spontaneously when one or more students are on placement in a particular work setting. Often the questions students ask have the effect of making experienced practitioners think again about their practice. For example, a student may ask: 'Why do you do it in this way?', only for the experienced worker to think: 'Yes, good question: why *do* we do it this way?'

Using enquiry and action learning (EAL)

EAL is an approach to learning that has been adopted on some professional training courses (see, for example, Parsloe 1996). It replaces traditional approaches to the curriculum with one based on an action-learning perspective. Taylor (1996: 83) describes the approach in the following terms:

> Lectures and seminars on discrete disciplines have been replaced by a problem-based learning approach where the 'study-unit' is the focal point for learning. A study unit lasts on average for two weeks and is built around a case scenario drawn from practice. Topics for the study units are determined by course planners with input from students about their learning needs. Students decide which aspect of the scenario to work on according to individual or group learning needs. Study unit work is the core of the course. It is supplemented by about two lectures a week on theoretical frameworks, two workshops a term on aspects of anti-discriminatory practice, and a skills development programme.

Clearly this involves quite a radical departure from traditional strategies for teaching and learning, but would appear to bring the learning situation much closer to the realities of practice and the ethos of reflective practice.

Such problem-based approaches can also be used on a smaller scale, for example as part of staff development or team-building workshop. In my view, the main value of this perspective on learning is that it begins with practice and seeks to incorporate the knowledge base and values associated with it, thus bypassing the common problem of beginning with theory and trying to apply it to practice in a technical-rational way.

Balancing challenge and support

Reid (1994) draws on the work of Daloz (1986) to argue the case for promoting reflective practice through achieving a balance of challenge and support. Consider the following four permutations of challenge and support and the likely outcomes of each:

- *Low support plus low challenge*: is likely to contribute to low morale and possibly a lack of commitment;
- *Low support plus high challenge*: can easily produce an atmosphere of fear and thus encourage defensiveness;
- *High support plus low challenge*: runs the risk of leading to too 'cosy' an atmosphere and possibly complacency;
- *High support plus high challenge*: is clearly the most effective combination as it encourages learning through challenge while providing the supportive atmosphere which can give staff the confidence to take the risks involved in learning (see the discussion of 'Staff care' below).

This framework of balancing challenge and support can be seen as a helpful way of creating a positive atmosphere in which reflection and learning are both encouraged and supported. The exploration of what steps can be taken to achieve this balance of high support and high challenge is therefore an activity that should pay dividends.

Developing staff care

Staff who are overstretched and loaded down by excessive pressures are clearly not going to be in an advantageous position when it comes to capitalizing on opportunities to learn from experience. Indeed, in situations of high stress, experience of work may be so painful or difficult that reflection on it is unlikely to occur, given the negative effects that can arise from thinking about such pressurized circumstances. A strategy of 'non-reflection' may well be an important coping mechanism for many staff seeking to manage a high level of stress.

Clearly, then, stress is a very significant barrier to the development of reflective practice. A high level of stress is likely to lead to a low level of reflection. Steps taken to tackle stress through the development of staff care (Thompson *et al.* 1994a, 1996a) are therefore likely to have the added bonus of facilitating reflective practice. Indeed, the two processes – developing staff care and promoting reflective practice – can be mutually supportive, each contributing to the development of the other.

Conclusion

A key element of professionalism is the existence and use of a theory base – formal knowledge grounded in law, policy and relevant academic disciplines. On this basis, then, professional practice cannot realistically be founded on an 'I prefer to stick to practice' attitude. Even those who reject professionalism as a form of elitist separatism would be hard pushed to justify rejecting the underpinning knowledge base of human services practice.

In view of this, the polarization of theory and practice must be seen as a destructive and dangerous process – and one to be very much avoided. The need to take steps to narrow the gap between theory and practice is therefore a very significant and pressing one. At best, the polarization of theory and practice restricts opportunities for learning and developing advanced practice and, at worst, increases the potential for dangerous practice.

The time and effort needed to integrate theory and practice therefore constitute a significant and worthwhile investment. The strategies briefly outlined in this chapter can go some way towards making such a sound investment. However, these strategies are, of course, neither comprehensive in their coverage nor guaranteed of a successful outcome. None the less, they do offer a substantial baseline from which to begin, or continue, the process of integration, a process which needs to become established as part and parcel of everyday practice.

A recurring theme in terms of integrating thought and action is that of reflective practice. This is a very useful concept which acts as an effective bridge between theory and practice. While acknowledging the value of the 'high ground' of science and research, it recognizes that this is not enough on its own to guide and inform the 'swampy lowlands' of practice. It is necessary for practitioners to reflect on their practice and tailor the knowledge base to suit the particularities of a complex and uncertain world of practice. It is in this sense that skilled practice can be understood as a successful blend of artistry and science.

It is to be hoped that the discussions in this chapter have, to a certain extent at least, paved the way for developing this 'blend'. What will also be clear, I hope, is that reflective practice in particular, and relating theory to practice in general, are not simple, mechanical processes. Indeed, the whole debate about theory and practice is a very complex one. What this reveals is that best practice is premised on skills – not only direct practice skills, but also the skills necessary for managing this difficult process of integrating theory and practice to best effect.

This raises the question of the preparation staff need to develop these skills – the education and training required to equip staff to respond positively to the challenge of developing an informed and reflective practice. Chapter 6 seeks to address this question, but within the broader context of the debate as to whether education or training – or some combination of the two – is the more appropriate basis for professional practice. Indeed, the basic task of Chapter 6 is to explore how education and training can facilitate, or hinder, the integration of theory and practice.

Food for thought

- Consider the gap between theory and practice.
  - In your view, what factors contribute to causing or widening a gap between theory and practice?
  - What implications might a gap between theory and practice have for day-to-day practice?
  - What implications might such a gap have for theory development?
- Consider reflective practice.
  - What does this term mean to you?
  - In what ways is it relevant to your work?
  - How might you promote the development of reflective practice?
- Consider the integration of theory and practice.
  - How is 'integrating theory and practice' different from 'applying theory and practice'?
  - Which of the strategies for integration are you likely to use in your own work?
  - Can you think of any additional approaches that might work for you?

Education and training: human resource development

Chapter overview

- What are the differences between education and training?
- How are knowledge, skills and values important?
- What are the advantages and disadvantages of competence-based training?
- What is person-centred learning?
- Why is it important?

Introduction

An important theme to emerge from the discussions so far is the central role of learning. Without recognizing, and facilitating, a process of learning, the integration of theory and practice is likely to be severely hampered. It is therefore important for us to explore further the significance of learning and the ways in which it is promoted through education and training.

This chapter therefore explores a range of issues relating to education and training, both as an initial preparation for practice and as an ongoing process within a programme of staff development. If human services staff are to gain maximum benefit from drawing links between theory and practice, there need to be regular opportunities for exploring and debating ideas and considering their implications for practice. Similarly, there need to be opportunities for reflecting on practice, learning from mistakes and building on strengths. Consequently, education and training have a significant part to play in developing an informed and reflective practice.

Vocational education and training and, more broadly, human

resource development (HRD) are important concepts which are instrumental in not only enhancing our ability to relate theory and practice, but also creating an atmosphere and culture conducive to relating the two. They are therefore major themes in this chapter. Other important topics to be covered include competence-based training and assessment; knowledge, skills and values; meta-learning and person-centred learning. However, before addressing these issues, it is important to explore and clarify a basic tension, that between education and training.

Education or training?

There is a longstanding debate about which is the more appropriate basis of professional practice, education or training. This debate was particularly prominent in social work in the early 1980s:

> Two 'camps' have been established. On the one hand we have writers such as Martin Davies (1982) who argue that social work students should be *trained*. This implies a programme of studies geared towards actual practice skills. He denies the usefulness of including academic studies such as sociology within the syllabus of professional social work training courses. The other school of thought (cf. Sibeon, 1982) retorts that Davies's 'technicalism' is inappropriate. Sibeon argues that social work students should be *educated*. They should be intellectually equipped to be able to locate their practice within the context of social policy issues and broader societal concerns.
>
> (Thompson 1992a: 19)

Education is therefore seen as a broader process than training and one which encompasses a notion of critical awareness. Goddard and Carew (1989: 22) reinforce this view when they argue that:

> Social workers need education not training. You can train monkeys, dogs and pigeons, and you can even train trees to climb walls, but social workers need more than this, much more ... Social workers need to start explaining the intellectual complexities and challenges inherent in their roles in order to create a more sympathetic view of their practice, and a more accurate perception of a profession at the cutting edge of intellectual activity.

Training is geared towards equipping staff with the skills they need to meet the demands of their work. It tends to be task-focused and, to a large extent, specific to particular job requirements. Education implies a broader process in which learning goes beyond immediate requirements and locates work tasks and demands in a wider professional context in which autonomy and creative approaches are encouraged.

Education is characterized by two features which distinguish it from technical training:

1. *A research base*: students and professional practitioners are expected to engage with a knowledge base which derives from research – that is, from systematic academic inquiry.
2. *A critical perspective*: education encourages people not to accept situations at face value, not to take things for granted. That is, education encourages people to *question*.

Both of these are present in the education of human services staff but, interestingly, in different proportions. Nurse education strongly emphasizes the importance of research, due in no small part to the influence of the Briggs Report (1972), in which the role of research was stressed:

> We have been given ample evidence that in nursing and midwifery education insufficient attention is paid to research as a continuing activity. Nor is there enough emphasis on research as a prelude to innovation. Nursing should become a research-based profession.
>
> (Briggs 1972: 108)

The significance of research has since become well-established and is seen as an essential component in the process of becoming a 'knowledgeable doer'.

In social work education, by contrast, there is some emphasis on research but to a far lesser extent than in nursing. There is, however, a much clearer focus on the need to develop a critical perspective. Qualifying social workers must be able to demonstrate an understanding of discrimination and oppression in society and therefore have to develop a critical understanding of social processes and institutions. Social work's commitment to social justice provides fertile soil for developing a critical social perspective.

In view of these differing emphases, both professions can learn from each other – nursing leads the way in demonstrating the role and value of research, while social work has made progress in developing a critical perspective.

However, the distinction between training and education is one of emphasis, rather than absolute difference. Training and education may well be very different in their pure forms but, in the reality of equipping people to undertake professional practice, the two can and do overlap to a considerable extent. Perhaps a more helpful and appropriate concept which incorporates elements of both training and education is that of 'human resource development'. In one way, this is an unfortunate term, in so far as describing people as a resource does have a rather impersonal ring to it. However, the ideas lying behind the term are very positive and constructive, albeit not without their limitations. The term derives from human resource management, an approach to the management of staff in organizations which differs from conventional personnel management in a number of ways, notably in its basic premise that an organization's staff are its most important asset or resource. Human resource development is therefore an approach to vocational education and training which seeks to maximize the potential of the people in the organization (the human resource). Clearly, then, human resource development is an important issue which has implications for the integration of theory and practice. It will therefore have an important part to play in the discussions below.

Knowledge, skills and values

Human resource development is generally recognized as having three dimensions – knowledge, skills and values. Each of these has an important part to play in promoting and enhancing effective professional practice. Each also needs to be seen in relation to the other two and the complex patterns which arise when they interact. For example, well-developed skills rely on an appropriate knowledge base, and both influence, and are influenced by, an underpinning set of values.

The knowledge base underlying human services practice is an extensive one, as Figures 6.1 and 6.2 indicate, using nursing and social work as examples. Clearly, it would be unrealistic to expect staff to have an in-depth understanding of every aspect of their respective professional knowledge base. What is needed, therefore, is:

- a good basic grasp of the rudiments of the professional knowledge base;
- the ability to gain access to more specialist knowledge as and when required;
- an awareness of the boundaries and limitations of one's current level of knowledge so that these are not dangerously exceeded;
- a commitment to continuous professional development so that one's knowledge base continues to grow and remains up-to-date.

A helpful way of perceiving the use of professional knowledge is in terms of a continuum, ranging from a dangerous complacency which eschews the value of professional knowledge at one extreme, to 'paralysis by analysis' in which people are not prepared to act until

Theory and Practice of Nursing – values; concepts; ideologies; models; information systems; research methodology and application

Communication Processes – working with individuals, families, groups and communities from different racial and ethnic groups; intra- and inter-professional work; counselling skills.

Relevant Social and Behavioural Sciences – human social development and behaviour and social, community, political and economic studies across all age groups and sexes related to individuals, groups, cultures and communities.

Life Sciences Relevant to Nursing Practice – normal and disordered structure and function; the nature and causation of disease; aspects of microbiology and pharmacology and their application to care provision.

Professional, Ethical and Moral Issues – codes and dilemmas; boundaries and complementary nature of medical and nursing practice; patient advocacy.

Organizational Structures and Processes – theory and structures; statutory framework and provision; statutory, voluntary and private services; working with medical practitioners and others involved in care; working in teams; nurses' duties and responsibilities within established policies; access to, and use of, information; and preparation for managing nursing teams.

Framework for Social Care Provision and Care Systems – present provision of care services; theoretical framework for care and management of resources.

Figure 6.1 The knowledge base of nursing (UKCC 1988)

they know all that there is to know at the other. Clearly, neither extreme is helpful and there is a positive balance to be struck, a successful middle range in which knowledge is used appropriately and to good effect.

Despite the value of knowledge as a guide to action, knowledge alone is not enough. In addition to knowledge, we need *skills*, a set of abilities or capacities which help to equip us to undertake our professional duties. Such skills are many and varied and can be divided into a number of categories, as Figure 6.3 illustrates. In general, these skills relate directly to practice. Some, however, such as self-management skills, play a more indirect, but none the less significant, role. Other such 'indirect' skills are those involved in *relating* knowledge to practice and, in the process, learning from doing so. This introduces the notion of 'meta-learning', an important concept to which I shall return below.

Skill development depends, in part at least, on practice, and therefore on experience. However, experience in practising a skill does not in itself lead to skill *development*. Kolb's work on the learning cycle (as discussed in Chapter 1) helps us to understand that using a skill (concrete experience) will only produce learning if it is reflected upon, related to previous learning and understanding, and put into practice in an informed way. That is, skill development does not simply

Social Work: Purpose, Models, Methods, Settings and Theories

- the range of human needs, especially those of vulnerable, disadvantaged and stigmatized groups;
- the process of observation, assessment (including risk analysis), planning, objective-setting, implementation, review;
- models for practice, work with individuals, including children, families, groups and communities;
- knowledge of transcultural factors which affect clients' needs and social work practice;
- aims, methods and theories for practice: counselling, advocacy, negotiation, task-centred work, crisis intervention, family therapy, group living, social education;
- the community and organizational settings of practice;
- the framework for practice – social work as part of a network of social service, health, criminal justice and penal provision.

Values
- the origin and justification, meaning and implication of the values of social work;
- ethical issues and dilemmas in practice, including the conflict of interest and rights that occur within families;
- ethical issues and dilemmas, including the potential for conflict between organizational, professional and individual values.

Law: Statutory Duties, Powers and Legal Principles
- individual liberty, natural justice, legal rights, human rights;
- structure and processes of the courts, including legal services;
- the social function of the law;
- welfare rights, income support, housing benefit;
- major statutory responsibilities;
- detailed knowledge of legal requirements.

Applied Social Sciences

- theories of human growth and behaviour, physical and psychological development of children, adulthood, ageing;
- family life-cycles, loss and change, identity, personality;
- social, family and community structures; processes of structural oppression, race, class, gender, disability; the notion of ethnocentricity;
- social welfare, theories of welfare, comparative social policies; the relevance of social security, housing, employment, penal policy, equal opportunities, and race relations to the delivery of social services;
- health and social conditions, causes and effects of crime, mental illness, learning difficulties, alcohol and substance abuse, AIDS;
- demographic and economic trends, relevant social research findings, and their evaluation and implications for practice.

Organizational Context
- organizational and institutional theory and structures;
- the structures of central and local government, the criminal justice system, and other relevant statutory, voluntary and private bodies, and their interrelationships;
- the implications of political, economic, racial, social and cultural factors upon service delivery, financing services and resource analysis;
- change theory, internal organizational structures and processes;
- computer and information technology, data protection and access to information, as relevant to social work practice.

Figure 6.2 The knowledge base of social work (CCETSW 1991)

happen – it can be helped or hindered by other factors, not least our own attitude towards the use of such skills.

At its simplest level, we can either entrust skill development to luck and assume that it will take place spontaneously, or we can take a more active approach towards such development by seeking out means of

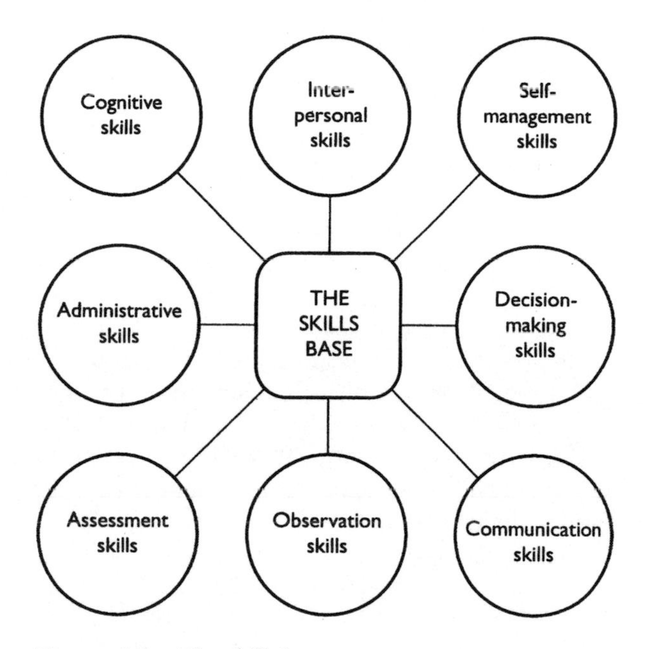

Figure 6.3 The skills base

maximizing the enhancement of skills and abilities. This latter approach is more consistent with reflective practice, as it implies a process of reflecting upon our actions in order to maximize both their effectiveness and the scope for learning from them.

An active approach to skill development is one which reflects the positive use of the concept of the 'locus of control'. Some people recognize the degree of control they have over their circumstances – they have an *internal* locus of control – whereas others play down the amount of influence they have and see control as *external* to them. The locus of control – external or internal – as perceived by the individual, will have a considerable impact on skill development in general and, in particular, on the skills involved in managing pressure and stress (Thompson 1996).

It is argued that perceived control over important areas of one's life is an important part of coping with pressure and stress. The 'locus' of control can be seen as either internal, in which case we have a positive view of how much control we have over our circumstances, or external, in which case we tend to attribute events to factors beyond our control and thus marginalize the part we play in determining our own circumstances. Andrisani and Nestel (1976, cited in Thompson *et al.* 1994a: 25) show:

> . . . 'internals' to be more successful in work, in terms of pay, promotion and job satisfaction, compared with their 'external'

counterparts. Individuals who see themselves as having more control over their lives are therefore more likely to cope with the pressures they face.

Such individuals are also more likely to be successful in skill development, as they will more fully recognize the active part they can play in enhancing their skills. This is one example of how skill development is not simply a matter of 'practice makes perfect'. An informed and reflective approach, that is one premised on the integration of theory and practice, has much more to offer. Relating theory to practice applies to skills as well as to knowledge.

The third dimension of human resource development is that of *values*. As we saw in Chapter 4, this places us in the realm of philosophy. The question of teaching a set of values is a complex, intricate and thorny one, as it exposes the risk of replacing education with indoctrination. It is beyond the scope of this book to address these issues in any depth. It is important to note, however, that any non-positivist approach to human resource development must take account of values. The question, therefore, is not *whether* to teach values, but *how*.

In order to avoid indoctrination, it is important that critical thinking is encouraged so that learners do not passively accept the teaching or other experiences they encounter. There is a need to engage critically with learning so that staff become active and creative learners, rather than 'well-trained robots'. This is a point to which I shall return later in relation to competence-based assessment.

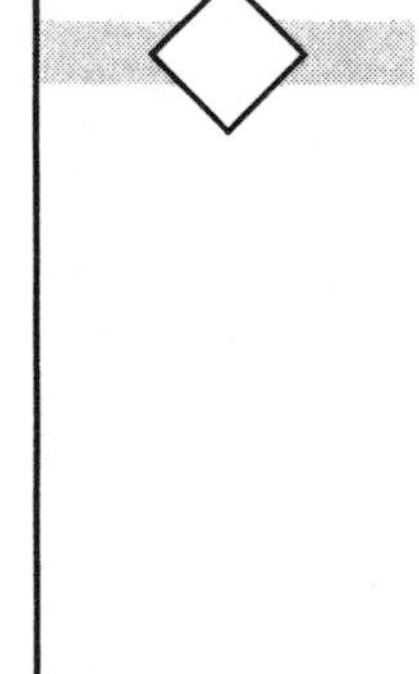

Practice Focus 6.1

Jenny was looking forward to her tutor's visit so that she could talk about the progress she had been making on her placement. Indeed, the tutor was delighted to learn of the major steps forward Jenny had made in her practical work. Discussion centred on the excellent progress made and Jenny was asked whether she could identify any changes that had contributed to the significant improvement. Without hesitation, she replied that there was one thing she felt had made a major difference. She described a lecture she had attended at which the 'locus of control' was discussed. She commented that understanding this concept had helped her to realize she had been defeatist about changes that needed to be made in her life, seeing them as beyond her control. That lecture had planted a seed which led to Jenny switching from an external locus of control to an internal one. This had given her confidence and brought about an improvement in a whole range of practice skills – organizational, time management and assertiveness.

Novak and Gowin (1984: xi) are critical of approaches to adult learning which concentrate primarily on changes in behaviour, rather than broader or deeper changes:

> . . . for almost a century, students of education have suffered under the yoke of the behavioral psychologists, who see learning as synonymous with a *change in behavior*. We reject this view, and observe instead that learning by humans leads to a *change in the meaning of experience*. The fundamental question . . . is, How can we help individuals to reflect upon their experience and to construct new, more powerful meanings?

This emphasis on meaning is characteristic of a phenomenological approach in which subjectivity and values are important factors to consider. Human resource development therefore needs to go beyond a focus on objective behavioural change to take account also of subjective changes in meaning and perspective. Values are clearly a central part of this, as they provide, by their very nature, a framework of meaning – they are a key part of each individual's *Weltanschauung*.

A theme underpinning all three dimensions of human resource development is, as noted earlier, that of the *person*, the sense of self which acts as a filter and fulcrum for our interactions with the outside world. It is the focal point for the dialectic of subjectivity and objectivity, the point of contact between the individual and the social world.

By recognizing the person as a central feature of human resource development, we also begin to recognize the key role of self-awareness or, as Gambrill (1990) puts it, 'self-knowledge'. She emphasizes the importance of clear thinking in making clinical judgements and then goes on to argue that:

> Clear thinking may become compromised by a lack of self-knowledge. Self-knowledge includes familiarity with resources and limitations of reasoning processes, as well as knowledge of strengths and limitations that influence decision making. In addition to limitations of knowledge, there are also attitudinal obstacles that compromise the quality of reasoning. These include carelessness, lack of interest in having a carefully reasoned position on a matter, a wish to appear decisive, and a vested interest in a certain outcome.
>
> (Gambrill 1990: 349)

Gambrill's focus is on the effects of self-knowledge on reasoning, but the same argument can also be applied more broadly to the use of theory in general. Awareness of one's own strengths, weaknesses and characteristic patterns is significant in relation to:

- *Knowledge*: as noted in Chapter 3, the facts do not 'speak for themselves'. Knowledge therefore has a strong subjective element within it.
- *Skills*: many of the skills involved in the human services are people skills, that is they involve 'use of self' – a reliance on our personality as a tool for helping to achieve our aims (Thompson 1996).
- *Values*: although established sets of values do exist (for example, religious, cultural and political), values are also very much a personal issue.

Self-awareness is therefore an important component of professional development, a key aspect of the 'personal foundation of experience':

> What the learner brings to the experience has an important influence on what is experienced and how it is experienced . . . The learner possesses a personal foundation of experience, a way of being present to the world, which profoundly influences the way it is experienced and the emotional content of the experience and the meanings which are attributed to it.
>
> (Boud and Walker 1990: 63)

There is, of course, also a social and political foundation of experience which needs to be considered. This is an issue which will feature in the discussion of person-centred learning later in this chapter.

Competence-based training: for and against

In the 1980s, the notion that training should be linked directly and explicitly to competence requirements gradually became dominant. A major step in this direction came with the introduction of national vocational qualifications (NVQs, or SVQs in Scotland) with explicit statements of the expected competencies to be demonstrated before a qualification could be awarded. This approach, while not universal, has become widespread and very influential.

For some, this development is seen as a major advance in vocational education and training, a significant improvement on traditional approaches. For others, however, this development is seen as a bureaucratic nightmare and a distortion of good practice in human resource development. My aim here is not to attempt to resolve this tension but, at a more modest level, to explore some of the key elements within this tension and consider their implications for relating theory to practice. I shall tackle this by outlining what I see as some of the main strengths and weaknesses of competence-based training.

A major strength of this approach is that the primary focus is on outcomes, a demonstrated capacity to perform effectively in terms of a particular task, skill or set of tasks and skills. This helps to avoid the situation where a member of staff has been exposed to a high-quality training input but, for whatever reason, the outcome has not been successful in terms of learning. A further advantage deriving from this is that, where training inputs are not of a high quality, this should become more apparent than was previously the case. Consequently, competence-based training has the potential to facilitate quality assurance and improved standards as far as training provision is concerned.

Having clear, predefined targets to aim for is also a strong point in terms of:

- reducing (but not eliminating) the part played by personal preferences in determining who has achieved competence and who has yet to achieve it;
- removing much (but not all) of the vagueness and confusion over what constitutes competent professional practice;
- recognizing and rewarding existing levels and areas of competence;
- reducing the anxiety and uncertainty over the criteria by which candidates will be judged;
- being transferable – success in one geographical area can be more readily recognized in another area if a candidate should move.

A significant advantage also is the recognition, implicit in this approach, that work-based learning extends far beyond attending training courses. That is, it is an approach premised on development, rather than simply training, as it recognizes the valuable learning opportunities presented in day-to-day practice (Thompson and Bates 1995).

There are, then, clear advantages to adopting a competence-based approach to training and assessment. However, it would be naive in the extreme to assume that benefits can be gained without also incurring costs. That is, the advantages need to be weighed against the disadvantages.

One such disadvantage is the complexity of detail which can be required in order to demonstrate competence. This leads many people to see this approach as unnecessarily bureaucratic and unduly time-consuming. The spirit of learning can be lost in the letter of competency detail. A further aspect of this is the tendency for competency statements to be worded in quite a jargonistic and inaccessible way. Ironically, this seems to have arisen in an attempt both to be precise and to cover a wide range of situations and circumstances.

The issue of losing the spirit of learning also applies more broadly than the phrasing of competence statements. One danger is that candidates lose track of a creative process of learning and focus narrowly on the predefined targets. This can lead people to focus on achieving *basic* competence, rather than *maximizing* learning. This is reflected in the fact that the term 'candidate' tends to be used, rather than 'learner'. In this way, the approach can be seen to be self-limiting.

Another criticism is that a reliance on predefined competencies is too standardized and does not, or cannot, take account of the wide variety of contexts in which practice takes place. This reflects the theoretical roots of the competence approach in behaviourist psychology with its focus on measurable, observable phenomena and a relative neglect of contextual factors. Field (1993: 47) refers to the work of Prior (1989) on this subject:

> Prior suggests that inappropriate attempts to promote assessment practices based on a behaviourist psychology have been so widespread because behavioural changes are easy to record and quantify, enabling managers to believe that they can account for what it is that they do. They cannot because of the unpredictability of social contexts and learning.

This echoes my earlier comments about the role of meaning in learning. Learning is not just about changing behaviour, it also involves a change in meaning or perspective. There is both a subjective and an objective dimension to learning, but an NVQ-style approach overemphasizes the objective at the expense of the subjective.

Field goes a step further by drawing a parallel between competence-based training and 'Fordism', the process by which industrial development broke down workers' skills into component parts so that productivity could be increased and the power of skilled workers decreased:

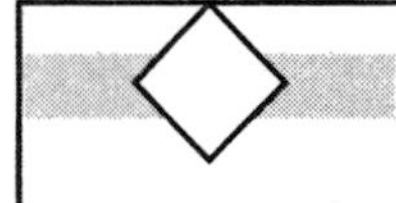

Practice Focus 6.2

Right from the start of his placement, Tony was only too aware that he had to demonstrate a number of predefined competences if he was to pass the course. This put him under a lot of pressure and, in the early stages of the placement in particular, his thoughts were dominated by the competences, a fact which actually held back his progress.

It was only at the point where he realized that this was happening that he could begin to learn. Up to that point, his anxiety to meet the competence requirements was actually preventing him from doing so. Fortunately, once he realized what had been holding him back, he was able to relax and focus on his learning needs. By doing so, he gave himself the space he needed to make significant progress and therefore had little difficulty in demonstrating his competence.

> Competency based assessment, in its present form, threatens to become the new Fordism of the education system. The proliferation of competency specifications and the increasing precision with which competences are stated parallels the 'parcellization' of the work-force and the labour process. As competences are differentiated more finely, so it becomes more and more possible to narrow the scope of initiative and field of responsibility of each individual in her work.
>
> (Field 1993: 48)

There is, therefore, a danger that such an approach will encourage 'skilled robots', rather than 'knowledgeable doers'. That is, this approach offers the advantages of a *training* ethos, but at the expense of the advantages of a perspective premised on the broader principles of *education*.

Whether an approach which draws on the benefits of competence-based training without compromising the principles of education can be developed, remains to be seen. This is a major challenge now facing HRD professionals, both within the human services and more broadly within the HRD community. This also entails a challenge for the learners themselves – to be able to maximize learning despite the constraints inherent in the current training ethos.

The strong influence of competence-based training also raises a number of issues for developing practice grounded in theory and values. While recognizing, and capitalizing upon, the benefits of a competency approach, we must be careful not to be seduced by it and thereby lose sight of its pitfalls and limitations. In particular, we need to remember that:

- Competences are very much in keeping with technical rationality. We also need to be in tune with the uncertainty and messiness of the 'swampy lowlands'.
- The standardized nature of competences can encourage a uniform approach and, in so doing, discourage creativity and imagination.
- What counts as competent practice is predefined. Practitioners, too, must have a say in what constitutes good practice, rather than simply accept it as given. That is, we need to adopt a *critical* approach.
- The competence-based approach recognizes the importance of underpinning knowledge but offers little guidance in how it can be used. Therefore, working towards achieving competences will not, in itself, facilitate the integration of theory and practice.

Clearly, then, the competence-based approach is by no means a panacea. As with training-based approaches in general, both its value and limitations need to be seen in the broader context of education, with an emphasis on critical reflection and self-directed learning.

Person-centred learning

An important distinction frequently drawn in the adult education literature is that between pedagogy and andragogy. The former is a term traditionally used to refer to teaching both children and adults, although literally it refers to children only. Andragogy, by contrast, refers specifically to adults and is therefore used to describe approaches to education and training which are particularly appropriate for adults. Referring to the work of Knowles (1978), Squires (1993: 92) comments:

> The word 'pedagogy' refers, strictly speaking, not to teaching but to the teaching of children . . . While Knowles does not suggest that there is a clear cut distinction between children and adults as learners, he does argue that teaching based on andragogical assumptions is appropriate to people in their late teens and beyond. The simple antithesis between pedagogy and andragogy has caught the imagination of many who work in adult education . . . It is worth pointing out, however, that Knowles is somewhat ambiguous about identifying andragogy solely with adult education; in some cases he presents it as a more enlightened approach to teaching younger age groups as well.

It is also worth pointing out that the derivation of the term andragogy is also commonly misunderstood – it refers to the education of *men*, rather than adults, and so gender is a significant dimension of this issue as well as age (Humphries 1988). Indeed, the gender dimension of adult learning is one that has tended to be neglected.

One major reason for seeking to go beyond pedagogy is that the education of children is, traditionally at least, teacher-centred. The aim of theorists such as Knowles is to seek to make adult education learner-centred, in the sense that the learner:

- is involved in defining his or her own learning needs;
- can influence the design and/or delivery of the curriculum through a process of consultation and negotiation;
- is actively involved in learning, for example through discussion or other forms of participation;
- is responsible for his or her own learning.

The concept of learner-centred education is one which is usually applied to formal learning situations such as courses. In such situations, the primary focus is, of course, on *learning*. However, the concept can be applied more broadly to take account of situations where learning can and does occur, but where learning is not the primary focus, that is, professional practice. Rogers (1961, quoted in Gardiner 1989: 56) comments on the importance of learner-centred education in terms which do not relate solely to formal learning opportunities:

> It seems to me that anything that can be taught to another is relatively inconsequential and has little or no significant influence on behaviour . . . the only learning which significantly influences behaviour is self-discovered, self-appropriated learning . . . [and] such self-discovery learning, truth that has been personally appropriated and assimilated in experience, can not be directly communicated to another . . .

Rogers's views here seem to be very close to those of Kolb in relation to the learning cycle. That is, learning derives from the interaction of the individual with the learning environment – it is not simply a matter of one person communicating knowledge to a group of others. Learning does not, therefore, simply occur in formal learning situations such as courses.

The term 'student-centred' learning is one that is commonly used but, clearly, the process of learning extends far beyond being a student. It is for this reason that I prefer the term 'person-centred learning'. This term also has the effect of emphasizing that learning is very much about personal experience – although, as I shall argue below, there is also a wider social and political dimension to consider.

Learning is a complex matter involving a range of factors. However, one recurring theme is the importance of recognizing learning as a *self-directed process*. As Mezirow (1981: 21) comments:

> Although the diversity of experience labeled adult education includes any organized and sustained effort to facilitate learning and, as such, tends to mean many things to many people, a set of standards derived from the generic characteristics of adult development has emerged from research and professional practice in our collective definition of the function of an adult educator. It is almost universally recognized at least in theory, that central to the adult educator's function is *a goal and method of self-directed learning*. Enhancing the learner's ability for self-direction in learning as a foundation for a distinctive philosophy of adult education has breadth and power. It represents the mode of learning characteristic of adulthood.

This does not mean that the learner is on his or her own in pursuing learning. Clearly, HRD staff have a key role in facilitating learning in terms of helping to create an atmosphere conducive to learning and helping to remove obstacles to learning, actual and potential. Other learners also have a part to play. To argue that learning should be self-directed is not to argue against collaborative or mutually supportive learning.

A crucial point to note in relation to self-directed or person-centred learning is that, without it, the integration of theory and practice is severely hampered. Person-centred learning allows people to *own* theory, to see knowledge and frameworks of understanding as useful and relevant to their concerns. Without this, there is a danger that staff will feel alienated from theory; they will see it as a matter for other people and not as a basis for their own practice. Person-centred learning can help to dispel myths about theory and practice:

> There are myths that surround theory development. Some of these are related to who could and should develop theories. One of these myths is that 'idea people' are 'ivory-tower types of individuals', that only extremely intelligent people can develop theories. Another myth is that there are theoreticians and there are practitioners; the former cannot practice and the latter cannot theorize.
>
> (Meleis 1991: 173–4)

These myths represent artificial barriers which can be dismantled so that theorists, educators and practitioners can be brought closer together in a spirit of shared endeavour.

An important concept with regard to person-centred learning is that of 'meta-learning' or, as Evans (1990) puts it, 'deutero-learning'. This refers to the process whereby learning becomes self-perpetuating – that is, whereby we learn how to learn:

> Learning to learn, or what *Bateson* (1973) calls deutero-learning, is a higher order conceptual skill whereby students may discover how it is they develop their practice and what inhibits this development. *Kolb et al.* (1979) and *Gardiner* (1989) have both developed explanatory models and methods of analysis which students can use to begin to discover how they best learn, and to adjust their strategies. Students also need to examine possible blocks to learning and to question their assumptions about the learning process.
>
> (Evans 1990: 31)

Evans sees this as an important skill in so far as it promotes continued learning beyond the point of qualification. That is, it acts as the basis of continuous professional development.

Gardiner (1989: 136) describes a three-stage model of learning, leading to meta-learning:

> *STAGE ONE is a surface-reproductive conception of learning, characterized by a predominant focus on the content of what is to be taught and learnt (i.e. facts or procedures) . . . [The] deeper conception of learning (STAGE TWO) is characterized by a focus on the process of learning (i.e. an active-constructive search for meaning from experience) . . . STAGE THREE conceptions of learning are characterized by a focus on meta-learning, and learning to learn* (i.e. being able to use and

evaluate qualitatively different approaches for different learning tasks).

This is clearly very consistent with Kolb's notion that we are responsible for our own learning (as discussed in Chapter 1) and therefore need to take an active, rather than passive, approach to learning. If learning is to be person-centred, it also has to be person-led, in the sense that the individual needs to take the initiative in making learning happen. As Abercrombie (1965: 41) puts it:

> There seem to be two main tasks in training for the professions: the task of passing on to the student an increasingly large and complex body of knowledge which it is necessary for him to master before he can practise his profession, and that of *preparing him to continue to learn, to adapt his skills to changing conditions, and even initiate change himself, to be inventive or creative.* (emphasis added)

However, while there is some considerable justification for placing a major responsibility for learning on the shoulders of the learner, we must also counterbalance this by recognizing the other factors that have an influence on learning, in particular the sociopolitical dimension.

Space does not permit a detailed analysis of these issues, but they are worthy of note none the less. The process of learning is a many-sided one and therefore one which interrelates with a wide range of social and political factors. These include:

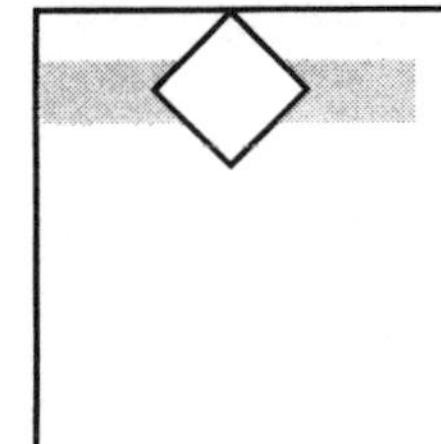

Practice Focus 6.3

Val had attended a number of in-service training courses over the years but it was one particular course that made all the difference for her. At the end of a course on community care, she was given an 'Action Plan for Learning' form to fill in. On this she was asked to identify: (1) what learning needs the course had revealed for her and (2) what steps she could take to meet those needs. This 'action plan' could then act as the basis for her future learning.

At first, Val saw little value in doing this. However, when she returned to work and discussed the plan with a colleague, she began to see how it could act as a focus for developing her knowledge and skills and act as a bridge between training and practice. Once she began the process, she appreciated how helpful and productive it could be and this increased her enthusiasm still further. She was moving away from the 'osmosis' approach to learning towards one based on 'meta-learning'. That is, she was learning how to take control of her own learning.

- *Gender*: a well-documented feature of sexism is its tendency to discourage high self-esteem in women and to encourage passivity. This can be seen to produce differential experiences of learning for women and men.
- *Race/ethnicity*: similarly, the pressures and hostilities inherent in racism can make for very different experiences of learning for people from ethnic minorities (see, for example, Rosen 1993). It is also important to consider issues of cultural diversity and ethnic sensitivity.
- *Age*: a common fallacy is the belief that older people are not able to learn. This is an example of ageism and one that we need to guard against. This is an attitude that can also be internalized by older people themselves and thereby act as a barrier to learning.
- *Class*: again, internalized expectations of achievement can be significant:

  > Although we experience barriers as internal – 'I can't possibly do that' or 'I don't want to do that' – they often arise from external influences which impacted on us at an earlier time and which left us feeling disempowered or de-skilled or inhibited. When we were treated as working-class boys who 'should' have low expectations of life, rather than as the particular individuals whom we were, we internalized the external oppression and censored our own aspirations.
  >
  > (Boud and Walker 1993: 81)

- *Language*: although English is a dominant language, we must remember that for many people in the English-speaking world, English is not their first language. Operating through the medium of a second language can be a significant barrier to learning and can place members of linguistic minorities at a disadvantage.
- *Organizational culture*: some organizations have a culture or ethos which encourages, supports and facilitates learning, whereas others have a culture which discourages, hinders or obstructs learning. This is an important issue I shall address in Chapter 7.

Addressing the social and political dimensions of learning is, of course, not an alternative to addressing the personal dimension – the personal needs to be understood in the context of the sociopolitical. There is a dialectical relationship between the subjective life-world of the individual and the objective context of social and political life – each needs to be understood in relation to the other. Ironically, then, an adequate understanding of person-centred learning must go far beyond the individual and take account of wider factors, a perspective entirely consistent with the principles of existentialism outlined in Chapter 4.

Conclusion

Developing human resources is recognized as a central part of a successful organization and effective professional practice. Vocational education and training therefore plays a pivotal role, particularly in relation to issues of theory and practice. This chapter has explored some of the key issues which arise in this respect, although clearly these are not the only ones. From an examination of human resource development in relation to the integration of theory and practice, a number of important points emerged, and it is worth repeating some of these by way of summary:

- Education and training are terms often used interchangeably. Education, however, is a wider concept than training and incorporates the notion of critical reflectivity.
- Human resource development (HRD) is a concept which incorporates both education and training and is based on the premise that a range of learning opportunities exist in professional practice in general and not simply on courses.
- HRD has three main dimensions: knowledge, skills and values. The three are interrelated and should not be seen in isolation. Learning is a continuous process involving all three elements and the dialectical interactions between them.
- Competence-based training and assessment has benefits, but also costs and limitations. We need to be cautious about adopting this approach wholesale. A more critical and balanced perspective is called for.
- HRD needs to be premised on person-centred learning, as this facilitates theory–practice integration and encourages staff to own their own learning.
- Person-centred learning, however, does not imply a neglect of wider social and political factors or the organizational context of learning.

There is now a considerable body of literature relating to adult education theory and human resource development. None the less, there is still considerable scope for the development of our understanding of these complex issues. We are still very much at the beginning of our investigations into this important aspect of human action and interaction.

However, our present level of understanding does allow us to challenge and dispel some of the myths relating to learning and the use of theory and practice. It is to be hoped that what we have learned so far about these processes can help to build confidence in tackling the issues and, in so doing, overcome many of the fears and fantasies that unreasonably stand in the way of maximizing both learning and the integration of theory and practice.

An important aspect of achieving maximum progress in these matters is the nature of the organizations in which we work and, in particular, their cultures. It is for this reason that the concept of organizational culture is one to be addressed in Chapter 7.

Food for thought

- Consider education and training.
  - In what ways is an *educational* approach necessary for your work within the human services?
  - In what circumstances is a *training* approach appropriate or helpful?
  - What would you see as the dangers of confusing the two or failing to recognize their differences?
- Consider competence-based training.
  - What problems might you encounter (or have encountered) in trying to demonstrate competence?
  - How might a competence-based approach help someone to learn?
  - How might it hinder learning?
- Consider person-centred learning.
  - What do you understand by 'person-centred learning'?
  - What do you see as its advantages?
  - How could you maximize the opportunities for person-centred learning?

The adventure of theory

Chapter overview

- Why is the organizational context important?
- What is a learning organization?
- Why is continuous professional development important?
- In what way is the practitioner also a theorist?
- How do we make the most of theory?

Introduction

Working in the human services involves a range of tasks and duties which are onerous, demanding and challenging. However, such work can also be immensely rewarding and satisfying. It is in this sense that such work can be described as an 'adventure' – a high level of demands upon us and high stakes, but also high rewards, potentially at least. This is not to romanticize human services work, but rather to set it in context – a context in which an ill-informed and ill-considered approach will not help to meet the challenges or achieve the rewards. The use of theory is therefore an important part of this adventure.

Furthermore, the process of relating theory to practice can be seen to be a form of adventure in its own right. Once again, high demands go hand in hand with high rewards. Integrating theory and practice to maximum advantage is challenging and fraught with difficulties, but also offers considerable potential benefits in terms of:

- improved levels of practice;
- increased opportunities for job satisfaction;

- a basis from which to justify decisions made and actions taken;
- continuous professional development.

The understanding, insight and knowledge that can be gained from relating theory to practice is, in itself, a major reward and one that justifies the commitment of time and energy required. For all these reasons, then, it is important that barriers to the integration of theory and practice are removed as far as possible. It is for this reason that the organizational context, and how it can help or hinder theory–practice links, needs to be addressed.

The organizational context

The context in which theory is related to practice is significant in a number of ways. In particular, the organizations staff work for can be very influential both directly and indirectly. A key concept in this respect is that of 'organizational culture'. Johanssen and Page (1990: 79) define culture as:

> Values, beliefs and customs of a group or type of people. In a company or corporation, its culture is demonstrated by its *management style*, including the degree of autocracy or participation practised . . . and the expectations of employees.

Organizations develop characteristic patterns and expectations which tend to have a very powerful influence on the staff who work within them. Such a culture can become firmly established and thereby create a dominant set of norms. These become so ingrained that new members of the organization need to be 'socialized' into the culture – they need to 'learn the ropes':

> Organizational culture is the *pattern of basic assumptions* that *a given group* has *invented, discovered, or developed in learning to cope* with its *problems of external adaptation and internal integration*, and that have *worked well enough to be considered valid*, and, therefore, *to be taught to new members* as the correct way to *perceive, think, and feel* in relation to those problems.
>
> (Schein 1992: 237)

The dominant culture within an organization can be a positive and constructive one, or it can be negative and destructive, a barrier to good practice. Where the latter applies, staff can be demotivated and frustrated by an atmosphere of negativism and cynicism, a problem which can ultimately lead to burnout (Thompson *et al.* 1994a). Indeed, a negative culture can create a spirit of helplessness, as Bate (1992: 214) points out:

> . . . people in organizations evolve in their daily interactions with one another a system of shared perspectives of 'collectively held and sanctioned definitions of the situations' which make up the culture of these organizations. The culture, once established, prescribes for its creators and inheritors certain ways of believing, thinking and acting which in some circumstances can prevent meaningful interaction and induce a condition of 'learned helplessness' – that is a psychological state in which people are unable to conceptualize their problems in such a way as to be able to resolve them. In short, attempts at problem-solving may become culture-bound.

In terms of integrating theory and practice, a culture characterized by negativity and helplessness will stand in the way of a positive practice premised on critical reflectivity. An organization which gives its staff a message of cynicism and low expectations will generate an atmosphere of low morale and will make a commitment to improving professional practice all the more difficult to achieve (Thompson *et al.* 1996b). A negative culture is therefore a serious barrier to integrating theory and practice, as it relies on routine standard responses to problems and situations, rather than reflection, critical analysis or creativity. Such a culture reduces stimulation, interest and job satisfaction and, in turn, the absence of these factors contributes to a negative atmosphere, thus making a negative culture a self-perpetuating process. What reinforces this process is the tendency for negative cultures to be *defensive*, to discourage risk and innovation. Breaking this destructive cycle is therefore an uphill struggle.

Practice Focus 7.1

Lynn was the officer-in-charge of an elderly people's home which had to close down as part of a reorganization of services. Consequently, she was redeployed to run another of the authority's homes where the previous officer-in-charge had retired. Lynn did not approach her new job with enthusiasm, as she was still feeling very sad about the closure of her previous home.

However, she soon had to change her approach as she was unhappy with the negative atmosphere and felt that her own lack of 'sparkle' was only making the situation worse. She was concerned about the cynical and defeatist attitudes which were commonplace among the staff. She recognized the existence of a negative culture, which was getting in the way of learning, creativity, job satisfaction and, of course, high-quality practice. Lynn therefore had to put her own feelings of disappointment and upset about her enforced job change aside and set about the task of creating a more positive and constructive atmosphere.

From this point of view, developing reflective practice is not simply an individual responsibility but, rather, a collective one. A commitment to improved standards of practice involves staff working together to promote a positive organizational culture and to challenge elements of negativity. Without this being a collective endeavour, the individuals who make the required efforts face an unnecessarily difficult struggle. However, a negative culture is by no means a feature of all organizations. Indeed, many organizations have a very positive and constructive culture, some having managed to transform a negative culture into a positive one. An important concept in this regard is that of the 'learning organization' (Garvin 1993; Schein 1993). As Roderick (1993: 13) puts it:

> The concept of 'The Learning Organisation' has . . . evolved over time, to the point where it now represents a coherent approach to maximising human potential in the service of organisational effectiveness. The key insight is that the capacity to learn individually and therefore organisationally, is an asset with huge survival value.

In recent years, many organizations have adopted a deliberate policy of becoming a learning organization, and this involves taking certain identified steps towards maximizing learning opportunities, both *within* the organization (for the individual) and *for* the organization (as a whole). Roderick (1993: 13) spells out in more detail what this entails:

> **Learning organisations do:**
>
> - take every opportunity to learn both from experience and in general at individual, group and corporate level
> - experiment with new ways of organising work and new ways of learning both within and outside the organisation
> - establish a climate in which learning from each other is actively supported
> - use the training function to facilitate the development and learning of all employees
> - see a key role for managers as facilitators
> - develop structures which encourage two-way communication as a means of promoting learning and development
> - encourage questioning, experimentation and exploration of new ideas at all levels
> - remove barriers and blockages to learning in both the individual and the environment
> - encourage and foster continuous learning and self-development in all employees
> - think about how to learn as well as what to learn.

Learning organisations do not:

- use command and control as the dominant method of management
- rely almost exclusively on formal conventional training as the primary source of learning and development within the organisation
- assume that past success is the key of future success
- take the view that the workforce is essentially passive and therefore incapable of autonomy and self-regulation
- take the view that new blood is the only means of achieving adaptive change in the belief that the existing workforce is too old to learn
- hold the belief that advanced information and manufacturing technologies are sufficient in themselves to guarantee success.

Developing a learning organization represents a strategy of culture change. It involves a concerted effort to change the values and assumptions dominant within an organization. Such a change of culture is not a simple matter and requires a major commitment of time and energy over an extended period of time. It is not an undertaking that can be taken lightly or one that can be entered into by only a minority of staff – it requires a whole-hearted commitment on a collective basis.

The culture of the organization in which we work is clearly a significant influence on the ways in which values, knowledge, ideas and actions will be integrated and interrelated. An organization's culture, and indeed the organizational context more broadly, can be instrumental in either helping or hindering staff in their efforts to develop reflective practice and integrate theory and practice.

Continuous professional development

This is a concept we encountered earlier. It refers to an approach to work characterized by a commitment to 'lifelong learning', an attitude of mind which guards against complacency and constantly seeks out new sources of learning and professional development. As such, continuous professional development (CPD) is an essential component of the 'adventure of theory'. It is also a widely recognized professional expectation, as exemplified by the UK Central Council for Nursing, Midwifery and Health Visiting (UKCC):

> As a registered nurse, midwife or health visitor, you are personally accountable for your practice and in the exercise of your professional accountability, must . . . maintain and improve your professional knowledge and competence.
>
> (UKCC 1992: 1)

CPD has a major contribution to make to high standards of practice in terms of:

- keeping up to date with changing circumstances and requirements;
- maintaining an openness to new ideas and new perspectives;
- adopting an approach based on critical reflectivity;
- maintaining an open mind in order to guard against prejudice and discrimination;
- providing an ongoing source of stimulation and motivation;
- a series of opportunities for mutual support and shared learning;
- a basis for teamwork and team development;
- a safeguard against burnout.

A further positive dimension of CPD is that it is 'infectious', in the sense that one person's commitment to CPD can rub off on others and act as a source of interest, stimulation and enthusiasm. The adventure of theory is one that can – and should – be shared by everyone. It is a starting point for a basis of shared endeavour and learning.

The Institute of Personnel and Development (IPD) provide a useful overview of what CPD is and what it is not:

> CPD is:
>
> - The integration of learning and work.
> - Recognising we operate in a rapidly changing world and that by developing ourselves we may influence these changes.
> - Owning and managing our own development.
> - Developing ourselves through an extremely wide range of activities – not simply off-the-job training . . .
> - Evaluation of learning – but you have to be strong enough to do it yourself!
> - Learning from things that went well and maybe not so well.
> - Planning to keep learning . . . continually
>
> **Emphasis is on the outcomes and not attendance.**
>
> It is:
> - what did you learn?
> - how do you plan to apply this learning?
>
> CPD is not:
>
> - what learning event did you experience?
> - about writing an exhaustive list of things I should have done
> - attending courses and doing nothing as a result of being there
> - checking off hours like 'brownie points'
> - 'big brother' creating paperwork
> - filling in forms for IPD.
>
> (IPD 1996)

CPD can be seen as an antidote to a traditional view of training and development as a means of addressing incompetence, an activity reserved for those who need it in order to overcome inadequacies in performance. CPD recognizes that training and development and, more broadly, learning and the integration of theory and practice are important concerns for all staff.

The practitioner as theorist

In addressing the question of the adventure of theory, it is worth considering the notion of the practitioner as theorist. This derives from the work of George Kelly (1955) and his theory of 'constructive alternativism'. Kelly's work falls broadly within the tradition of phenomenology, with its emphasis on meaning and perception. The basic premise of Kelly's work is that reality is not 'given', in any absolute sense, it has to be interpreted or *constructed*.

The term constructive alternativism refers to the fact that there is a wide range of alternative constructions of reality. Different people will interpret the world in different ways. We make sense of the world in our own way and thus create our own reality. (There are strong parallels here with the dialectic of subjectivity and objectivity discussed in Chapter 4.) In this way, we are constantly constructing our reality by making sense of the world as we encounter it.

In order to aid us with this task, we develop what Kelly referred to as 'personal constructs'. A construct is a bipolar dimension we use to make distinctions and to categorize people, things, events or ideas. Examples of constructs would be: good–bad, friendly–hostile, interesting–boring. Kelly argues that we use sets of constructs as a framework for understanding our experiences by identifying patterns of similarities and differences.

A major implication of Kelly's model is that the individual is a theorist, in the sense that he or she develops, and constantly adjusts and modifies, a framework for understanding – that is, a theory. Kelly therefore describes individuals as 'scientists'. For example, he sees both psychologists and their clients as groups of scientists:

> Both may be regarded as scientists, if you please, as well as men, for both seek to anticipate events. Both have their theories in terms of which they try to structure the onrush of occurrences. Both hypothesise. Both experiment. Both observe. Both reluctantly revise their predictions in the light of what they observe on the one hand, and the extent of their theoretical investment on the other.
>
> (Kelly 1980: 24)

This is an important analogy, as it portrays practitioners (and, indeed, all people) as theorists in the sense that practice involves:

- making sense of experience;
- making predictions/anticipating;
- relating events to a pre-existing body of knowledge;
- forming hypotheses and testing them out;
- using general principles to develop a framework of understanding;
- addressing conflicts between one's own views and those of others.

The analogy of the practitioner as theorist is therefore a very apt one which helps us understand how theory and practice interlink. It also casts light on the fallacy of theoryless practice in so far as it illustrates the extent to which ideas and actions are subtly interwoven. As such, it helps to dispel myths which act as a barrier to the optimal integration of theory and practice.

Kelly's ideas were proposed and developed as a means of explaining how we each construct our own sense of reality through a system of 'constructs'. It was not specifically intended as a 'theory of relating theory to practice', but succeeds in that respect none the less. It provides us with a useful picture of the personal construction of reality, the personal perceptions and cognitions which give us a basis from which to think, feel and act. However, once again we need to see such personal, individual matters in the broader context of the sociopolitical factors which have a bearing on them. That is, in addition to the personal construction of reality, we need to consider the *social* construction of reality.

Berger and Luckmann (1966) emphasize the importance of social factors in shaping our personal sense of reality. They use the term 'typifications' to describe what, in Kelly's terms, could be seen as collectively shared constructs, ideas or beliefs, which are commonly ascribed to within a cultural group or across a society. Such typifications act as basic building blocks of the social construction of reality. Typifications include social expectations in terms of how people should behave with regard to, for example, gender roles, age, occupation or class, and are therefore very significant aspects of social life. As Berger and Luckmann (1966: 47–8) comment:

> The social reality of everyday life is thus apprehended in a continuum of typifications ... Social structure is the sum total of these typifications and of the recurrent patterns of interaction established by means of them. As such, social structure is an essential element of the reality of everyday life.

When we conceive of the practitioner as theorist, we must also address the sociopolitical factors of power, social divisions, social processes and so on. We must be wary of adopting an individualist perspective which pays insufficient attention to the sociopolitical context.

Incorporating sociopolitical factors into our understanding of the practitioner as theorist raises a number of important issues and implications:

- Our 'social location' (that is, where we fit into society in terms of our sex, class, age and so on) will influence the way we perceive the world and respond to it.
- Our patterns of thinking and feeling are culture-specific. If we do not make the effort to practise in an ethnically sensitive way, we are likely to act in an ethnocentric way and thereby contribute to racism.
- In our 'theorizing', vested power interests in society will push us in certain directions and constrain us from pursuing others. That is, *ideology* can be seen to operate and certain sanctions, for example being labelled 'radical' or 'extremist', will be applied to people who express particular viewpoints.
- There is a need to work collectively so that ideas can be shared, perspectives broadened and networks of mutual support established.

A central theme to emerge from a consideration of the sociopolitical context is the need, once again, to develop an approach premised on critical reflectivity, an approach which replaces myth with knowledge, assumption with analysis and tacit acceptance with critical awareness. The practitioner does indeed act as a theorist – theory and

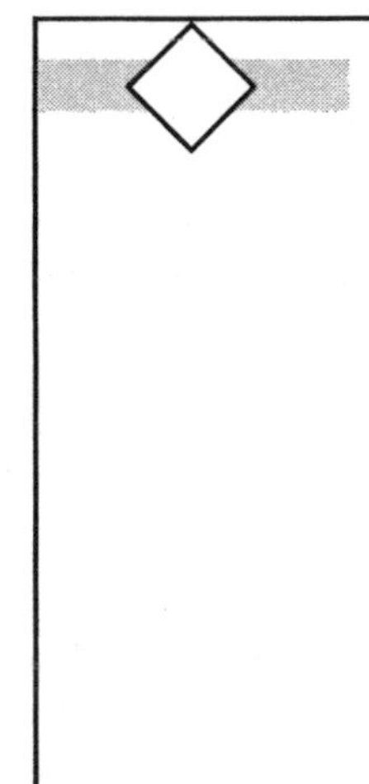

Practice Focus 7.2

When Shirley became a health visitor, one of the first things to strike her about her new duties was the significance of social factors such as poverty, deprivation and racism. In her previous experience as a nurse, she had had no contact with people in their homes and so she had not developed a picture of just how significant such factors are in people's lives.

Seeing the poor housing of so many of her clients and seeing the cumulative effects of years of reliance on state benefits, she was able to see health in much broader terms than before. It was only now that her course lectures on sociology came to life and meant something to her in concrete, practical terms. She began to realize that the demands of her new job meant that she would have to take much more account of social factors in future, as these were clearly such a central feature of her clients' experience.

practice *are* integrated, as I have argued at various stages. However, what I have also argued is that, for such integration to be at an *optimal* level, it needs to be critical, reflective and committed to challenging discrimination and oppression.

Dealing with uncertainty

A further key element in the adventure of theory is the ability to deal with uncertainty and the problems and challenges it presents. As Gambrill (1990: 328) comments:

> How uncertainty is handled influences the quality of clinical decisions. It can be denied or ignored; that is, clinicians can (and often do) act as if a higher degree of certainty is warranted than is the case. Choice of this option may result in overlooking alternative, more accurate accounts. Recognizing the uncertainty involved in making clinical decisions and taking steps to reduce it is the approach recommended here . . . Acknowledging uncertainty does not mean that clinical decisions are not made; it means that they are made in spite of uncertainty, taking whatever steps possible to decrease it.

However, it is not simply a matter of seeking to reduce uncertainty – this is not always possible. It is also a matter of accepting, and learning to cope with, the demands of working within a context of uncertainty: 'The role of uncertainty needs to be appreciated. Some aspects of uncertainty can be reduced but the primary task is to learn to cope with uncertainty and indeed help others to learn to do so' (Thompson 1992b: 35).

There is a parallel here with Schön's (1983) rejection of technical rationality as a basis for the swampy lowlands of practice. No matter how hard we try, we cannot expect professional practice, with all its complexities, subtleties and contingencies, to fit neatly into the orderly parameters of technical rationality. House's (1979) argument that teaching is best seen as a craft, rather than a technology (the former being based on tacit knowledge, experience and apprenticeship, the latter on explicit knowledge and principles), can be applied more generally to other forms of professional practice.

It is a question of developing the skills necessary to cope with the 'messiness' of human services practice. This is a significant dimension of the adventure of theory – seeking to meet the challenge of uncertainty or, to use the existentialist term, the contingency of being.

In this context, it can be seen that relating theory to practice is not a matter of finding the 'right answers' in a predefined body of knowledge but, rather, generating answers through a creative process of critical reflectivity. In this way, relating theory to practice is to be seen as a process, rather than an event. The adventure of theory entails managing that process to maximum effect.

The first step in this direction is to accept the significant role of uncertainty and recognize its *existential* nature. This can be illustrated by reference to the very uncertain enterprise of child protection in which the concept of risk plays such an important role:

> The concept of risk is a major one in child protection as is the recognition that there can be no 'guarantees', no cast-iron answers as to what is the appropriate way forward. Struggling to cope with such complexities, tensions and dilemmas of choice and responsibility – of human freedom – are *existential* issues. It is an existential process about which conventional wisdom tells us little or nothing.
>
> (Thompson 1992b: 11–12)

And it is here that we encounter a paradox. In recognizing uncertainty as an essential dimension of practice, we need to find ways of coping with it. However, there can be no simple, formula solutions which offer a certain way forward. The way forward, in terms of coping with the indeterminacy of practice, is one which

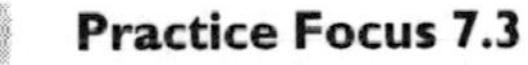

Practice Focus 7.3

A social services office was the setting for Lyndon's final placement before completing his social work training. Lyndon had done well on the course and felt very confident. He coped well with the caseload he was allocated, but each week he spent a day as the duty social worker and this caused him major difficulties. As the duty social worker, he encountered an enormous range of different problems, needs and circumstances. Due to this diversity, there was no way of predicting what the next problem was likely to be.

It was this unpredictability which created tremendous uncertainty for Lyndon, and this was something he found very difficult to deal with. At one point, his anxiety about this constant uncertainty was having a serious effect on his confidence and was causing him to make a lot of basic mistakes. Fortunately, Lyndon's practice teacher was very skilled and experienced at dealing with student problems. She was able to help him get over his anxiety and adopt a more confident and flexible approach to duty work. Her intervention succeeded in allowing Lyndon to realize that trying to reduce uncertainty is not the only way of coping with it. He had begun to learn the lesson that working with people inevitably involves working with a degree of uncertainty.

needs to be actively managed and negotiated, an ongoing and ever-present challenge – the challenge of the adventure of theory.

Rising to this challenge involves achieving *authenticity* by discarding the bad faith which would have us deny the significance of uncertainty and take comfort in the false security of technical rationality and positivism. Achieving authenticity involves consistency of thoughts, feelings and actions – a genuine integration of theory and practice. A key part of this, as we saw in Chapter 4, is *le vécu*, lived experience, for it is only by being in touch with lived experience that we can tackle the complexities of practice, without the bad faith of formula answers.

Making it happen

In order to draw on the benefits of the adventure of theory, it is necessary to seek the optimal integration of theory and practice. In effect, this has been the primary theme of the book – the value of using theory to guide practice and practice to test theory. In view of this, what needs to be done now is to revisit and summarize the main points presented throughout the book in order to pull together the main threads of my argument.

This will serve a dual purpose. On the one hand, it will act as a concluding summary of the main themes and issues and, on the other, it will provide the basis of an action plan for 'making it happen' – translating the adventure of theory into a practical reality.

I shall present a number of key points in outline form, although clearly this will not amount to a comprehensive list. The range of issues covered has been broad, varied and complex, and so it is to be hoped that a restatement of the main themes will help to provide an overview of this rather tangled web.

It is also important to emphasize that it is neither possible nor desirable to present a set of 'answers' or simple steps to follow. The challenge is to be able to wrestle with the immense complexities of theory and practice and for each of us to find our own way forward – to tailor the cloth to fit the circumstances we face, rather than look for ready-made answers in this book or anywhere else. What follows, then, is intended as a guide to the process of developing our own ways forward, and not as a substitute for it.

1. *Both learning and relating theory to practice are active processes.*
   This point derives from Kolb's theory of the learning cycle and emphasizes that the individual is responsible for his or her own learning *and* for integrating theory and practice. Although others such as managers, educators and so on have a part to play in promoting and facilitating informed practice, it is practitioners who have responsibility for 'making it happen'.

2. *Professionalism is based on knowledge.*
   The knowledge base underpinning practice is the basis of professionalism as part of a process of seeking to maximize effectiveness. In this context, professionalism can be seen not as a form of elitism, but as a commitment to high-quality practice.

3. *Good practice must be anti-discriminatory practice.*
   Sociological theory sensitizes us to the divisions and conflicts in society and the discrimination and oppression these engender. This helps us to recognize that our practice must also be sensitive to these issues. If we are not, our practice can at best condone oppression, and at worst reinforce and exacerbate it.

4. *Rejecting theory has many costs.*
   Expressing a preference for 'sticking to practice', as if theory had no value or relevance, is not without its costs. If we turn our backs on theory, we run the risk of practising in an uninformed, haphazard way; colluding with discrimination and oppression; being unable to evaluate practice systematically; missing opportunities for job satisfaction and staff development; and so on.

5. *The mystique of theory and anti-intellectualism are two major barriers to the optimal integration of theory and practice.*
   A common problem is for theory and practice to become 'polarized'; an artificial and unhelpful wedge is driven between them. This tends to manifest itself in two ways – theory can be mystified and thus distanced from practice, or theory is devalued and rejected as having little or no relevance to practice. Both these extremes stand in the way of informed practice.

6. *Positivism is an inadequate basis for the human services.*
   The inappropriate attempt to apply the methods and principles of the natural sciences to social science has bedevilled the development of theory and methodology in social work and health care. Spurious attempts to gain scientific status in this way are doomed to failure, in that they seek to exclude a very important dimension of human existence – that of subjective experience.

7. *Research has an important role to play but also has limitations.*
   There are two harmful extremes to be avoided here. On the one hand, it is important that research is not dismissed as an academic irrelevance. On the other, however, research also needs to be subjected to critical scrutiny, rather than accepted unquestioningly at face value. Finding the constructive balance between the two extremes is the basis of research-minded practice.

8. *Philosophy provides a framework of ideas and values to act as an overarching framework.*
   Specific theories tend to focus on a narrow range of phenomena to be explained and, in many cases, the role of values is marginalized, either implicitly or explicitly. Philosophy, by contrast, adopts a much wider focus and explicitly incorporates a value position. It is therefore well suited to the wide and complex demands of the rigours of practice. It is important, therefore, that practitioners do not shy away from philosophical matters.

9. *Technical rationality leaves practitioners ill-equipped to deal with the 'swampy lowlands of practice'.*
   Professional practice takes place in a context of complexity, conflict, uncertainty and change. It is therefore characterized by 'messiness' and does not fit neatly into theoretical schemata based on technical rationality. A broader and more flexible perspective is called for. Theory needs to fit practice, rather than practice being distorted to fit a particular theory.

10. *Dialectical reason offers a more appropriate basis for practice than analytical reason.*
    Analytical reason involves breaking situations down into their component parts so that we can begin to understand their interrelationships. While this has considerable value, it also has limitations. Dialectical reason transcends these limitations by accounting for change and movement by reference to the interaction of conflicting forces. This provides a fuller understanding of the change and conflict inherent in the human services.

11. *Existentialism offers a sound philosophical basis for professional practice.*
    Existentialist philosophy provides a value base and explanatory framework well suited to the humanistic basis of social work and health care and the inherent uncertainty of such work. In particular, the concept of *authenticity* – the rejection of self-deception or 'bad faith' – is a central one. An authentic practice is one in which staff fully recognize that they are responsible for their own actions and do not seek excuses in some form of determinism.

12. *Reflective practice is the starting point for informed practice.*
    In order to maintain and enhance standards of professional practice, it is essential that practitioners *reflect* on their practice that is, engage in a critical and reflective dialogue with the situations in which they operate. Reflective practice avoids the

pitfalls of a routine, uncritical practice which can do more harm than good.

13. *Practice is inevitably based on some form of theory – the task is to make this process as effective as possible.*
The notion of a practice which does not rely on a knowledge base or a theoretical perspective can be seen to be a fallacy. Theory and practice are therefore necessarily integrated. However, an uncritical, non-reflective integration of theory and practice is of relatively little value. What needs to be promoted is the *optimal* integration of theory and practice, a practice which maximizes the use and value of theory, rather than taking it for granted.

14. *Education offers a broader perspective than training.*
Professional practice needs to be supported by training so that knowledge and skills can be improved and updated. However, an approach which simply *trains* staff is self-limiting. What is also needed is an approach to human resource development premised on *education*, in which critical analysis and self-directed learning are promoted.

15. *Human resource development is premised on knowledge, skills and values.*
In order to maximize the human potential of staff working in the human services, it is necessary to focus on three particular areas: the knowledge base which informs practice, the skills which characterize good practice and the values which underpin it.

16. *Competency-based training has benefits but also has limitations.*
Vocational training has, in recent years, become heavily influenced by competency-based assessment of training outcomes. While this has certain advantages, it also has serious limitations, and so there is a danger that an over-reliance on such an approach will stand in the way of maximizing learning.

17. *The most appropriate form of learning is person-centred learning.*
Where staff take responsibility for their own learning and engage in self-directed learning, positive outcomes can be maximized through the tailoring of experiences to learning needs, high levels of motivation and reward, and the development of 'meta-learning' – the ability to 'learn how to learn'.

18. *Professional practice is characterized by uncertainty.*
Working in a health care or social work context brings us face to face with a number of uncertainties. Professional judgement is necessarily characterized by risk and so the danger of 'getting it

wrong' is ever-present. While some degree of certainty and security has considerable appeal, practitioners need to face up to the reality of a practice in which uncertainty is never far away.

19. *The practitioner is also a theorist.*
As the work of Kelly (1955) indicates, practitioners address their work in a way which parallels that of the scientist, in terms of developing working hypotheses and testing them against experience. Although the process may not be as systematic or explicit as that of scientific investigation, practice does involve a process of making sense of experience in which we test our expectations against the actual situations we encounter.

20. *It is important to promote an attitude of continuous professional development.*
Working with people is complex, demanding and subject to constant change. There is a need, therefore, for staff to continue to learn, to continue developing knowledge and skills and to keep in touch with the new demands of practice. Continuous professional development is therefore not only an essential part of good practice, it is a source of stimulation, motivation and job satisfaction.

Conclusion

Working in the human services is neither simple nor straightforward. The demands and challenges of such work are often of major proportions and can test us to the limits. Given this context, it is important that staff are as well equipped as possible to meet these challenges.

Of course, no theory base can guarantee success in coping with the demands of practice. However, I hope that what this book has shown is that a systematic and imaginative use of theory can help to prepare for the rigours of practice and help us guard against the pitfalls that stand in the way of effective and appropriate interventions.

The efforts involved in optimizing the integration of theory and practice should therefore be seen as a worthwhile investment of thought, time and energy. In deciding whether or not we should make such an investment, we should consider the costs involved in not making such an investment. That is, the key question is not 'Can we afford to integrate theory and practice?' but, rather, 'Can we afford not to?'

Food for thought

- Consider the organizational context.
  - What aspects of organizations can prevent or lessen opportunities for learning?
  - What is a 'learning organization'?
  - What can individual staff do to contribute to developing a learning organization?

- Consider continuous professional development.
  - Why is such development so important?
  - How can you ensure you continue to learn?
  - How can you support others in learning?

- Consider making the most of theory.
  Of the principles listed in the chapter:
  - Which ones are likely to be easiest for you to implement?
  - Which are likely to be the most difficult?
  - Are there any other principles you can identify that relate to your work situation?

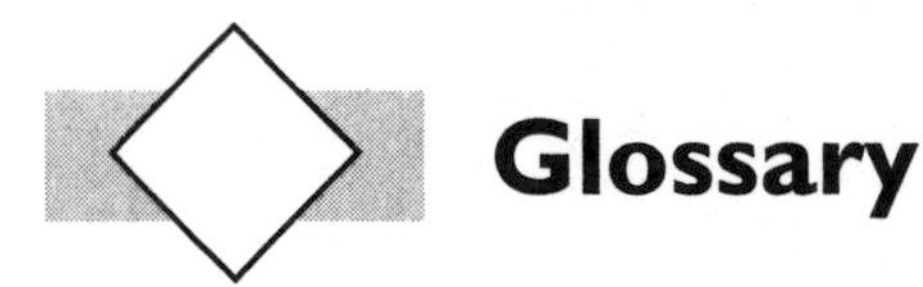

Glossary

Abstract conceptualization This is stage three of Kolb's learning cycle (*qv*). It refers to the process of mentally linking a new experience with our previous knowledge and experience in order to make sense of it.

Active experimentation This is stage four of Kolb's learning cycle (*qv*). It refers to implementing learning by behaving differently as a result of the understanding or insights gained through the process of learning.

Anti-discriminatory practice An approach to practice which recognizes the pervasiveness of various forms of discrimination and oppression and the need to ensure that these are i) taken into consideration when assessing situations, planning and implementing responses; and ii) countered wherever possible. See Thompson (1997) and/or Thompson (1998a).

Anti-intellectualism A tendency to devalue the contribution that theory and formal knowledge can make to practice. An anti-intellectual stance is one in which it is assumed that effective practice can be achieved without drawing on a knowledge base other than one's own experience or 'practice wisdom' passed on from one generation of workers to another. Such an approach fails to appreciate the significant role of theory and research in informing practice and falls foul of the 'fallacy of theoryless practice' (*qv*).

Authenticity A key concept in existentialism which refers to the absence of 'bad faith' (*qv*). An authentic existence is one in which the significance of freedom and responsibility are fully recognized and no attempt is made to deny or evade the fact that each individual is responsible for his or her own actions and their consequences.

Bad faith A tendency to deceive ourselves into thinking we are not responsible for our actions. This can take many forms, relating to biological, environmental or other forms of determinism. It is seen as a way of coping with the pressure of taking responsibility for ourselves by presenting factors over which we have control (our behaviour, for example) as if they were fixed and unchangeable. For example, sex offenders often claim that they 'could not help themselves' (see Thompson 1992b).

Competence-based training An approach to training and professional development which is based on the identification of 'core competencies', specific aspects of skills, knowledge and, to a lesser extent, values presumed necessary for the successful performance of duties in a particular post.

Once such competencies have been identified, training and subsequent assessment are expected to be geared towards them.

Concrete experience This is the first stage in Kolb's learning cycle (*qv*). Learning begins with a concrete experience, whether an experience specifically geared towards learning (attending a training course or reading a book, for example) or simply an experience as part of everyday life.

Constructive alternativism A theory developed by George Kelly (Kelly 1955) in which it is posited that people act as a form of scientist by developing their own hypotheses about social reality and testing these out through experience. Kelly argues that this is how we learn about society and our place within it. from this hypothesis-testing we develop 'bipolar constructs' – sets of opposites, such as 'friendly–unfriendly', 'safe–dangerous', 'pleasant–unpleasant', and subsequently use such constructs to develop further hypotheses.

Continuous professional development A commitment to continuing to learn and develop throughout one's career, rather than simply learn enough to work at a competent level and then abandon any further attempts to learn. Often abbreviated to CPD, this concept has been influential in encouraging organizations to make the best use of the human resources available to them through appropriate approaches to staff development.

Critical theory An approach to theory which emphasizes the need to recognize individual actions (human agency) in the broader context of social relations and institutions and the power relations on which they are based. A central theme is a recognition of the need to adopt a *questioning* approach to social reality, rather than accept it at face value.

Dedifferentiation A recognition of the arbitrary nature of boundaries between academic disciplines. This concept alerts us to the dangers of maintaining strict divisions between, say, psychology and sociology and the need to avoid unhelpful or unduly restrictive boundaries.

Dialectical reason A form of reasoning based on the dynamic interaction of conflicting forces. That is, it is recognized that one force or entity comes into conflict with another and, as a result of the interaction between the two, a new synthesis is produced. For example, in a team setting, one individual's wishes may conflict with those of another team member. This conflict may then result in a new synthesis – a new set of circumstances arising from the conflict. Thus, dialectical reasoning is characterized by conflict and change.

Discrimination A set of processes by which an individual or group receives unfair or less advantageous treatment, usually as a result of a social 'marker' such as class, ethnic group, gender, age and so on. One common consequence of discrimination is oppression (*qv*).

Eclecticism An approach to practice based on combining elements from different theories or theoretical traditions, generally in an uncoordinated way.

Enquiry and action learning An approach to professional training based not on traditional teaching methods, but focused rather on identified problems or case scenarios. The aim is to *integrate* theory and practice through activities that reflect the 'swampy lowlands' of practice, rather than the technical-rational approach of *applying* theory to practice.

Essentialism This is one of the four 'cardinal sins of theorizing'. It refers to the tendency to treat fluid, changing processes as if they were fixed entities incapable of change. For example, an essentialist view of selfhood would see identity as fixed and unchangeable rather than as a developing process.

Evaluation The activity of examining interventions (usually after they have been completed) with a view to identifying how effective they were; what was done well; what could have been done better; and what lessons can be learned (see Shaw 1996, 1997).

Existentialism A philosophy which emphasizes the important role of freedom in social life. It is based on the central notion that not only can each of us choose, but also we *must* choose, as to avoid choice is, in itself, a form of choice. Existentialism stresses the importance of recognizing how much control we have over our own actions and argues that we should be aware of the responsibility we carry for those actions.

Hermeneutics An approach to science and research which stresses the important role of interpretation and meaning.

Human resource development An approach to vocational education and training based on the principles of human resource management, particularly the notion that people are an organization's most important resource and therefore worthy of considerable investment in terms of learning and professional development.

Human services A range of occupations sharing the common theme of dealing with personal and social problems. This includes nursing and health care generally; social work and social care; youth and community work; probation and community justice; counselling, advocacy and mediation.

Ideographic theory Forms of theory which are concerned with describing and explaining specific, narrowly-defined sets of phenomena, as opposed to 'nomothetic' theories which seek to generalize findings from specific circumstances to account for a much wider range of phenomena.

Ideology A set of ideas which supports a particular set of power relations. For example, patriarchal ideology reinforces ideas about men's and women's respective roles in society and thereby plays a part in the maintenance of those role expectations.

Interprofessional learning Opportunities for learning created by different professional groups sharing training or other staff development activities, each group being able to benefit from the different perspectives the other groups bring.

Learning cycle A model of learning in which it is proposed that learning takes place through a cycle comprising four stages: concrete experience; reflective observation; abstract conceptualization; and active experimentation (*qv*). Stemming from the work of David Kolb and his colleagues, this approach has been influential in adult education settings and has emphasized the active nature of learning.

Learning organization A term used to describe the type of organization which invests heavily in promoting learning, not only through conventional training and development activities but also throughout the organization in whatever ways possible. This is a logical extension of the notion that an organization's staff are its most important resource. Such an important resource therefore needs to be developed to the full through continuous learning.

Lived experience (*le vécu*) This is an important term in existentialist philosophy which emphasizes the importance of theoretical perspectives presenting human existence as concrete, lived experience, rather than something abstract or unconnected with day-to-day reality.

Mentoring A form of personal or organizational support in which an experienced worker or manager acts as a guide and facilitator of learning for someone with less experience.

Model A step in the process of theory-building in which various pieces of information (or 'data') are organized into a pattern or picture so that their interrelationships can be identified. A model is therefore useful for describing a complex set of phenomena and paves the way for the next stage of theory-building – the development of an explanation for those phenomena.

Nomothetic theory See 'ideographic theory'.

Oppression 'Inhuman or degrading treatment of individuals or groups; hardship and injustice brought about by the dominance of one group over another; the negative and demeaning exercise of power. Oppression often involves disregarding the rights of an individual or group and is thus a denial of citizenship.' (Thompson 1997: 32–3)

Organizational culture A set of norms, values and assumptions taken for granted within a particular organizational setting, but none the less having a significant influence on the actions and attitudes of individuals and groups within that organization. In a way, an organizational culture represents the 'unwritten rules' of that organization.

Paradigm A 'family' of models or theories. A collective term for a number of related approaches which share a particular emphasis or set of premises – for example, various behavioural theories can be categorized under the heading of the 'behavioural paradigm'.

Person-centred learning An approach to personal and professional development which emphasizes the importance of starting with experience and seeking to integrate theory and practice, rather than try to 'apply' theory to practice as if theory were able to provide ready-made solutions.

Phenomenology Literally 'the study of perception', phenomenology is a philosophical perspective which emphasizes the role of interpretation and the construction of meaning. It is therefore concerned with the processes through which the objective social world is experienced by the individual at a subjective level.

Positivism An approach to science and research which stresses the need for 'objectivity' (in the sense of being value-free), precise measurement and the development of natural 'laws'. It is an approach that has been heavily criticized for being overly rigid and therefore unsuited to the complexities of social reality.

Power At its simplest, power is the ability to achieve what one intends. However, it is a very complex concept operating at different levels: personal, cultural and structural – see Thompson (1998a).

Problematic, the The subject-matter to be explained by a particular theory. Theories are attempts to develop explanations of particular phenomena or sets of phenomena. The focus of attention of a given theory is referred to as 'the problematic'.

Problematizing This is a process that can be used to develop reflective practice. It involves taking an aspect of everyday work or life – one that is straightforward and not problematic in any way – and looking at it from different angles to learn more about it (by getting beneath the veneer of what we normally take for granted and making it more *problematic*).

Professionalism A contested term, but one used in this book to refer to a commitment to high standards of practice based on i) clear and explicit values; and ii) a formal knowledge base incorporating the knowledge and experience of others over a long period and distilled in the professional literature and elsewhere.

Reductionism One of the four 'cardinal sins of theorizing', it refers to the tendency to reduce a complex, multilevel phenomenon (such as discrimination) to a single level explanation (such as personal prejudice or bigotry). As such, it is a form of oversimplification.

Reflective observation This is the second stage of the learning cycle (*qv*). It refers to the process of thinking about an experience, reflecting on it, so that we are then ready for the third stage (abstract conceptualization) of relating it to our existing experience or understanding.

Reflective practice An approach to professional practice premised on a critique of technical-rationality (*qv*). It presents practice as a process of wrestling with complex and 'messy' issues, rather than seeking ready-made solutions from theory, research, more experienced colleagues or elsewhere. It recognizes the value of theory and research as providing the 'cloth' from which practice solutions can be created, but emphasizes that it is the craft of the reflective practitioner which enables specific solutions to be tailored to the particular circumstances.

Reification One of the four 'cardinal sins of theorizing', it refers to the tendency to treat an abstract or generalized entity as if it were a concrete thing capable of decision-making and independent action. The statement that 'The poor have only themselves to blame for their predicament' is an example of reification. It assumes that people subjected to poverty ('the poor') form an entity that, in itself, can make decisions and take actions. It combines the actions of numerous individuals and groups over a long historical period and presents them as if it were simply a matter of a particular entity making a particular decision or acting in a particular way. Terms like 'the poor' are a shorthand but can often be treated as if they referred to a unified group which acts in a unified or coordinated way.

Research-minded practice An approach to professional practice which emphasizes i) the important role of research in informing practice; and ii) the dangers of neglecting or ignoring research studies relevant to our particular area of practice.

Routinized practice A dangerous form of practice where the need to assess situations and determine the most appropriate way of dealing with them is replaced by a tendency to deal with diverse situations in a uniform way. While routines have an important part to play in effective workload management, an over-reliance on them can lead to overly simple response to complex situations.

Staff care A set of organizational policies and practices geared towards i) protecting staff from the negative effects of stress in particular; and ii) supporting and valuing staff in general.

Technical rationality An approach to professional practice based on the (false) assumption that theory and research can provide formula solutions, direct procedures to follow or other such protocols that can be followed. This stands in direct contrast with reflective practice (*qv*).

Teleology One of the four 'cardinal sins of theorizing', this refers to the tendency to ascribe purpose or intentionality to phenomena inappropriately. For example, to argue that the 'purpose' of unemployment is to discipline the workforce (to make sure that workers are motivated to 'toe the line') is to fall foul of teleology. This argument implies that unemployment was deliberately designed for a particular purpose. It therefore confuses an historical outcome or effect (the existence of unemployment) with an assumed cause ('they' made it that way).

Theory A framework of ideas geared toward explaining a particular phenomenon or set of phenomena. Theories can be *formal* – for example, the ideas presented in textbooks, journals and so on – or *informal*, the often unacknowledged sets of ideas developed from experience and rarely recorded or identified explicitly as 'theory', but which none the less serve to explain the phenomena we encounter.

Theoryless practice The false assumption that practitioners carry out their duties without drawing on any particular theory or knowledge base. It is often characterized by comments such as 'I prefer to stick to practice'.

Values The things we attach value to, for example principles or ethics. Values are often to be found in formal 'sets of values', such as religious or political values. However, we also have our own personal values which may draw in part on formal value systems.

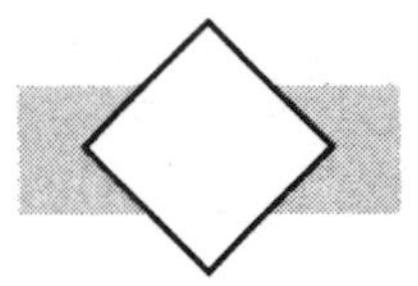

References

Abbott, P. and Sapsford, R. (1988) *The Body Politic, Health, Family and Society*, Unit 11 of the Open University Course, D211 Social Problems and Social Welfare, Milton Keynes, The Open University.

Abbott, P. and Sapsford, R. (eds) (1992) *Research into Practice: A Reader for Nurses and the Caring Professions*, Buckingham, Open University Press.

Abercrombie, J. (1965) 'The Nature and Nurture of Architects', *Transactions of the Bartlett Society* 2 (reproduced in Nias, 1993).

Andrisani, P.J. and Nestel, I. (1976) 'Internal/External Control as a Contributor to, and Outcome of Work Experience', *Journal of Applied Psychology*, 61.

Argyris, C. and Schön, D.A. (1974) *Theory and Practice*, San Francisco, CA, Jossey-Bass.

Aron, R. (1965) *Main Currents in Sociological Thought*, Vol. 1, Harmondsworth, Penguin.

Asch, D. and Bowman, C. (1989) *Readings in Strategic Management*, London, Macmillan.

Barnes, H. (1974) *Sartre*, London, Quartet.

Bate, P. (1992) 'The Impact of Organizational Culture on Approaches to Organizational Problem-Solving', in G. Salaman (ed.) *Human Resource Strategies*, London, Sage.

Bateson, G. (1973) *Steps to an Ecology of Mind*, London, Paladin.

Beauvoir, S. de (1972) *The Second Sex*, Harmondsworth, Penguin.

Benner, P. (1984) *From Novice to Expert*, London, Addison-Wesley.

Benton, T. (1981) '"Objective" Interests and the Sociology of Power', *Sociology*, 15(2).

Berger, P. and Kellner, H. (1981) *Sociology Reinterpreted*, Harmondsworth, Penguin.

Berger, P. and Luckmann, T. (1966) *The Social Construction of Reality*, Harmondsworth, Penguin.

Best, S. and Kellner, D. (1991) *Postmodern Theory: Critical Interrogations*, London, Macmillan.

Betts, K. (1986) 'The Conditions of Action, Power and the Problem of Interests', *The Sociological Review*, 34(1).

Bevan, D. (1998) 'Death, Dying and Inequality', *Care: the Journal of Practice and Development*, 7(1).

Billington, R. (1990) *East of Existentialism*, London, Unwin Hyman.

Birt, R. (1997) 'Existence, Identity and Liberation', in L.R. Gordon (ed.) *Existence in Black: An Anthology of Black Existential Philosophy*, London, Routledge.

Boud, D.J. and Walker, D. (1990) 'Making the Most of Experience', *Studies in Continuing Education*, 12(2).

Boud, D.J. and Walker, D. (1993) 'Barriers to Reflection on Experience', in D.J. Boud, R. Cohen and D. Walker (eds) *Using Experience for Learning*, Buckingham, Open University Press.

Boud, D.J., Keogh, R. and Walker, D. (eds) (1985) *Reflection: Turning Experience into Learning*, London, Kogan Page.

Boyne, R. and Rattansi, A. (eds) (1990) *Postmodernism and Society*, London, Macmillan.

Brake, M. and Bailey, R. (eds) (1980) *Radical Social Work and Practice*, London, Edward Arnold.

Briggs, A. (1972) *Report of the Committee on Nursing*, London, HMSO.

Buckenham, J.E. and McGrath, G. (1983) *The Social Reality of Nursing*, Balgowlah, Australia, ADIS Health Science Press.

Burr, V. (1995) *An Introduction to Social Constructionism*, London, Routledge.

Carter, J. (ed.) (1998) *Postmodernity and the Fragmentation of Welfare*, London, Routledge.

CCETSW (1991) *Rules and Requirements for the Diploma in Social Work* (Paper 30), 2nd edn, London, Central Council for Education and Training in Social Work.

Chamberlain, S., Crosher, I., Sherratt, N. and Woodward, K. (1990) 'Men and Women and Society: Tutor Notes', Milton Keynes, The Open University.

Chinn, P.L. and Kramer, M.K. (1991) *Theory and Nursing: A Systematic Approach*, 3rd edn, St Louis, Mosby Year Book.

Clamp, C. (1980) 'Learning Through Incidents', *Nursing Times*, 76(40).

Compton, B.R. and Galaway, R.R. (1979) *Social Work Processes*, Homewood, IL, Dorsey Press.

Corrigan, P. and Leonard, P. (1978) *Social Work Practice under Capitalism: A Marxist Approach*, London, Macmillan.

Cousins, C. (1987) *Controlling Social Welfare*, Brighton, Wheatsheaf.

Coutts-Jarman, J. (1993) 'Using Reflection and Experience in Nurse Education', *British Journal of Nursing*, 2(1).

Curnock, K. and Hardiker, P. (1979) *Towards Practice Theory: Skills and Methods in Social Assessments*, London, Routledge and Kegan Paul.

Curt, B.C. (1994) *Textuality and Tectonics*, Buckingham, Open University Press.

Daloz, L.A. (1986) *Effective Teaching and Mentoring*, London, Jossey-Bass.

Davies, M. (1982) 'A Comment on Heart or Head', *Issues in Social Work Education*, 2(1).

Department of Health (1988) *Protecting Children: A Guide for Social Workers Undertaking a Comprehensive Assessment*, London, HMSO.

Department of Health (1991) *Patterns and Outcomes in Child Placement*, London, HMSO.

Derrida, J. (1976) *Of Grammatology*, Baltimore, Johns Hopkins University Press.

Dewey, J. (1933) *How We Think*, Boston, MA, D.C. Heath.
Donald, J. and Hall, S. (eds) (1986) *Politics and Ideology*, Milton Keynes, Open University Press.
Douglas, T. (1986) *Group Living*, London, Tavistock.
Dunn, A. (1985) 'Foreword', in J. Salvage (ed.) *The Politics of Nursing*, London, Heinemann.
Equal Opportunities Commission (1987) *Women and Men in Britain: A Statistical Profile 1986*, London, HMSO.
Equal Opportunities Commission (1988) *Women and Men in Britain: A Research Profile 1987*, London, HMSO.
Etzioni, A. (1969) *The Semi-Professions and Their Organization*, New York, Free Press.
Evans, D. (1990) *Assessing Students' Competence to Practise*, London, CCETSW.
Everitt, A., Hardiker, P., Littlewood, J. and Mullender, A. (1992) *Applied Research for Better Practice*, London, Macmillan.
Eysenck, H.J. (1965) *Fact and Fiction in Psychology*, Harmondsworth, Penguin.
Feyerabend, P. (1975) *Against Method*, London, Verso.
Field, J. (1993) 'Competency and the Pedogogy of Labour', in M. Thorpe, R. Edwards and A. Hanson (eds) *Culture and Processes of Adult Learning*, London, Routledge.
Fish, D., Tuinn, S. and Purr, B. (1989) 'How to Enable Learning through Professional Practice. A Cross-Profession Investigation on the Supervision of Pre-Service Practice: A Pilot Study – Report Number One', West London Institute of Higher Education.
Foucault, M. (1977) *Discipline and Punish: The Birth of the Prison*, London, Allen Lane.
Foucault, M. (1979) *The History of Sexuality, Vol. 1: An Introduction*, London, Allen Lane.
Fox, N.J. (1993) *Postmodernism, Sociology and Health*, Buckingham, Open University Press.
Frankl, V. (1973) *Psychotherapy and Existentialism*, Harmondsworth, Penguin.
French, R. and Grey, C. (eds) (1996) *Rethinking Management Education*, London, Sage.
Further Education Unit (1988) *Learning by Doing*, London, FEU.
Gambrill, E. (1990) *Critical Thinking in Clinical Practice*, San Francisco, CA, Jossey-Bass.
Gardiner, D. (1989) *The Anatomy of Supervision*, Milton Keynes, Open University Press.
Garvin, D.A. (1993) 'Building a Learning Organisation', *Harvard Business Review*, July/August.
Giddens, A. (1993a) *New Rules of Sociological Method*, 2nd edn, Cambridge, Polity.
Giddens, A. (1993b) *Sociology*, 2nd edn, Cambridge, Polity.
Gilbert, N. (ed.) (1993) *Researching Social Life*, London, Sage.
Goddard, C. and Carew, R. (1989) 'Social Work: Mechanical or Intellectual?', *Social Work Today*, 19 January.
Gordon, L.R. (ed.) (1997) *Existence in Black: An Anthology of Black Existential Philosophy*, London, Routledge.

Gould, N. (1996) 'Introduction: Social Work Education and the "Crisis of the Professions" ', in N. Gould and I. Taylor (eds) *Reflective Learning for Social Work*, Aldershot, Arena.
Gould, N. and Taylor, I. (eds) (1996) *Reflective Learning for Social Work*, Aldershot, Arena.
Gray, C. and Pratt, R. (eds) (1990) *Towards a Discipline of Nursing*, London, Churchill Livingstone.
Griseri, P. (1998) *Managing Values: Ethical Change in Organisations*, London, Macmillan.
Grossberg, L. (1996) 'History, Politics and Postmodernism: Stuart Hall and Cultural Studies', in D. Morley and K.-H. Chen (eds) *Stuart Hall: Critical Dialogues in Cultural Studies*, London, Routledge.
Habermas, J. (1972) *Knowledge and Human Interest*, London, Heinemann.
Habermas, J. (1979) *Communication and the Evolution of Society*, Cambridge, Polity.
Hardiker, P. and Barker, M. (1991) 'Toward Social Theory for Social Work', in J. Lishman (ed.) *A Handbook of Theory for Practice Teachers*, London, Jessica Kingsley.
Harding, S. (ed.) (1987) *Feminism and Methodology*, Milton Keynes, Open University Press.
Heather, N. (1976) *Radical Perspectives in Psychology*, London, Methuen.
Heisenberg, W. (1958) *The Physicist's Conception of Human Nature*, London, Hutchinson.
Held, D. (1980) *Introduction to Critical Theory, Horkheimer to Habermas*, London, Hutchinson.
Hollinger, R. (1994) *Postmodernism and the Social Sciences*, London, Sage.
Hopkins, J. (1986) *Caseworker*, Birmingham, Pepar.
House, E. (1979) 'Technology Versus Craft', in P.H. Taylor (ed.) *New Directions in Curriculum Studies*, Brighton, Falmer Press.
Howe, D. (1987) *An Introduction to Social Work Theory*, Aldershot, Arena.
Hughes, B. and Mtezuka, M. (1992) 'Social Work and Older Women: Where Have Older Women Gone?', in M. Langan and L. Day (eds) *Women, Oppression and Social Work: Issues in Anti-Discriminatory Practice*, London, Tavistock/Routledge.
Hugman, R. (1991) *Power in Caring Professions*, London, Macmillan.
Humphries, B. (1988) 'Adult Learning in Social Work Education: Towards Liberation or Domestication?', *Critical Social Policy*, 23.
IPD (Institute of Personnel and Development) (1996) *Continuing Professional Development: A Guide to 'Doing' CPD*, IPD Merseyside, North Cheshire and North Wales Branch.
Jay, M. (1973) *The Dialectical Imagination*, London, Heinemann.
Johanssen, H. and Page, G.T. (1990) *International Dictionary of Management*, London, Guild Publishing.
Johnson, D.P. (1981) *Sociological Theory: Classical Founders and Contemporary Perspectives*, New York, John Wiley.
Kelly, G. (1955) *A Theory of Personality: The Psychology of Personal Constructs*, New York, W.W. Norton.
Kelly, G. (1980) 'The Psychology of Optimal Man', in A.W. Landfield and L.M. Leitner (eds) *Personal Construct Psychology, Psychotherapy and Personality*, New York, John Wiley.

Kempner, T. (1987) *The Penguin Management Handbook*, Harmondsworth, Penguin.

Knowles, M. (1978) *The Adult Learner: A Neglected Species*, 2nd edn, Houston TX, Gulf.

Koestler, A. (1964) *The Act of Creation*, London, Hutchinson.

Kolb, D.A. (1984) *Experiential Learning*, Englewood Cliffs NJ, Prentice-Hall.

Kolb, D.A. and Fry, R. (1975) 'Towards an Applied Theory of Experiential Learning', in C.L. Cooper (ed.) *Theories of Group Processes*, London, John Wiley.

Kolb, D.A., Rubin, I.M. and MacIntyre, J.M. (1979) *Organizational Psychology*, Englewood Cliffs NJ, Prentice-Hall.

Krill, D.F. (1978) *Existential Social Work*, London, Collier Macmillan.

Laing, R.D. (1967) *The Politics of Experience and the Bird of Paradise*, Harmondsworth, Penguin.

Langer, E. (1991) *Mindfulness*, London, HarperCollins.

Lash, S. (1990) *Sociology of Postmodernism*, London, Routledge.

Lecomte, R. (1975) 'Basic Issues in the Analysis of Theory for Practice in Social Work', PhD Thesis, Ann Arbor MI, Bryn Mawr College, the Graduate School of Social Work and Social Research.

Lendrum, S. and Syme, G. (1992) *Gift of Tears: A Practical Approach to Loss and Bereavement Counselling*, London, Routledge.

Lesnik, B. (ed.) (1997) *Change in Social Work*, Aldershot, Arena.

Lesnik, B. (ed.) (1998) *Countering Discrimination in Social Work*, Aldershot, Arena.

LoBiondo-Wood, G. and Haber, J. (1990) *Nursing Research: Methods, Critical Appraisal and Utilization*, 2nd edn, St Louis, Mosby.

Macdonald, G., Sheldon, B. and Gillespie, J. (1992) 'Contemporary Studies of the Effectiveness of Social Work', *British Journal of Social Work*, 22(6).

Mahon, J. (1997) *Existentialism, Feminism and Simone de Beauvoir*, London, Macmillan.

May, R., Angel, E. and Ellenberger, H.F. (eds) (1958) *Existence: A New Dimension in Psychiatry and Psychology*, New York, Basic Books.

McLellan, D. (1975) *Marx*, London, Fontana.

Meleis, A.I. (1991) *Theoretical Nursing: Development and Progress*, 2nd edn, New York, J.B. Lippincott.

Mezirow, J. (1981) 'A Critical Theory of Adult Learning and Education', *Adult Education*, 32(1).

Miles, R. (1989) *The Women's History of the World*, London, Paladin.

Mills, C.W. (1970) *The Sociological Imagination*, Harmondsworth, Penguin.

Morley, D. and Chen, K.-H. (eds) (1996) *Stuart Hall: Critical Dialogues in Cultural Studies*, London, Routledge.

Morrison, T. (1993) *Staff Supervision in Social Care: An Action Learning Approach*, London, Longman.

Nias, J. (ed.) (1993) *The Human Nature of Learning*, Buckingham, Open University Press.

Novak, J.D. and Gowin, D.B. (1984) *Learning How to Learn*, Cambridge, Cambridge University Press.

Oliver, M. (1983) *Social Work with Disabled People*, London, Macmillan.

Oliver, M. (1990) *The Politics of Disablement*, London, Macmillan.

Oliver, M. (1992) 'Changing the Social Relations of Research Production', *Disability, Handicap and Society*, 7(2).

Oliver, M. and Sapey, B. (1999) *Social Work with Disabled People*, 2nd edn, London, Macmillan.

Palmer, A., Burns, S. and Bulman, C. (eds) (1994) *Reflective Practice in Nursing: The Growth of the Professional Practitioner*, Oxford, Blackwell.

Parker, B. and Creasia, J.L. (1991) 'Theories and Frameworks for Professional Nursing Practice', in J.L.Creasia and B. Parker (eds) *Conceptual Foundations of Professional Nursing Practice*, St Louis, Mosby Year Book.

Parse, R.R. (1987) 'Paradigms and Theories', in R.R. Parse (ed.) *Nursing Science: Major Paradigms, Theories and Critiques*, Philadelphia, PA, W.B. Saunders.

Parsloe, P. (1996) 'Managing for Reflective Learning', in N. Gould and I. Taylor (eds) *Reflective Learning for Social Work*, Aldershot, Arena.

Pascall, G. (1986) *Social Policy: A Feminist Analysis*, London, Tavistock.

Pilalis, J. (1986) ' "The Integration of Theory and Practice": A Re-examination of a Paradoxical Expectation', *British Journal of Social Work*, 16(1).

Powell, J.H. (1989a) 'The Reflective Practitioner in Nursing', *Journal of Advanced Nursing*, 14.

Powell, J.H. (1989b) 'Reflection and the Evaluation of Experience: Prerequisites for Therapeutic Practice', in R. McMahon and A. Pearson (eds) *Nursing as Therapy*, London, Chapman and Hall.

Preston-Shoot, M. and Agass, D. (1990) *Making Sense of Social Work: Psychodynamics, Systems and Practice*, London, Macmillan.

Prior, L. (1989) 'Evaluation Research and Quality Assurance', in J. Gubrium and D. Silverman (eds) *The Politics of Field Research: Sociology Beyond Enlightenment*, Beverly Hills, CA, Sage.

Pugh, R. (1997) 'Change in British Social Work: The Lure of Postmodernism and its Pessimistic Conclusions', in B. Lesnik (ed.) *Change in Social Work*, Aldershot, Arena.

Rafferty, D. (1992) 'Implications of the Theory/Practice Gap for Project 2000 Students', *British Journal of Nursing*, 1(10).

Ramazanoglu, C. (1989) 'Improving on Sociology: The Problems of Taking a Feminist Standpoint', *Sociology*, 23(3).

Reid, B. (1994) 'The Mentor's Experience: A Personal Perspective', in A. Palmer *et al.* (eds) *Reflective Practice in Nursing: The Growth of the Professional Practitioner*, Oxford, Blackwell.

Roberts, J. (1996) 'Management Education and the Limits of Technical Rationality: The Conditions and Consequences of Management Practice', in R. French and C. Gray (eds) *Rethinking Management Education*, London, Sage.

Roberts, R. (1990) *Lessons from the Past: Issues in Social Work Theory*, London, Tavistock/Routledge.

Roderick, C. (1993) 'Becoming a Learning Organisation', *Training and Development*, March.

Rogers, C. (1961) *On Becoming a Person: A Therapist's View of Psychotherapy*, London, Constable.

Rojek, C., Peacock, G. and Collins, S. (1988) *Social Work and Received Ideas*, London, Routledge.

Rosen, V. (1993) 'Black Students in Higher Education', in M. Thorpe, R.

Edwards and A. Hanson (eds) *Culture and Processes of Adult Learning*, London, Routledge.

Sartre, J.-P. (1976) *Critique of Dialectical Reason*, London, Verso.

Sartre, J.-P. (1948) *Anti-Semite and Jew*, New York, Schocken.

Sayer, A. (1992) *Method in Social Science: A Realist Approach*, 2nd edn, London, Routledge.

Schein, E.H. (1992) 'Coming to a New Awareness of Organizational Culture', in G. Salaman (ed.) *Human Resource Strategies*, London, Sage.

Schein, E.H. (1993) 'How Can Organisations Learn Faster?', *Sloan Management Review*, Winter.

Schön, D.A. (1983) *The Reflective Practitioner*, London, Temple Smith.

Schön, D.A. (1987) *Educating the Reflective Practitioner*, San Francisco, CA, Jossey-Bass.

Schön, D.A. (1992) 'The Crisis of Professional Knowledge and the Pursuit of an Epistemology of Practice', *Journal of Interprofessional Care*, 6(1).

Seaman, C.H.C. (1987) *Research Methods: Principles, Practice and Theory for Nursing*, 3rd edn, Norwalk, CT, Appleton and Lange.

Shipman, M. (1988) *The Limitations of Social Research*, London, Longman.

Shaw, I. (1996) *Evaluating in Practice*, Aldershot, Arena.

Shaw, I. (1997) *Be Your Own Evaluator*, Wrexham, Prospects Publications.

Shotter, J. (1975) *Images of Man in Psychological Research*, London, Methuen.

Shotter, J. (1993) *Cultural Politics of Everyday Life*, Buckingham, Open University Press.

Sibeon, R. (1982) 'Theory-Practice Symbolizations: A Critical Review of the Hardiker/Davies Debate', *Issues in Social Work Education*, 2(2).

Sibeon, R. (1990) 'Comments on the Structure and Forms of Social Work Knowledge', *Social Work and Social Sciences Review*, 1(1).

Sibeon, R. (1991) *Towards a New Sociology of Social Work*, Aldershot, Avebury.

Sibeon, R. (1996) *Contemporary Sociology and Policy Analysis: The New Sociology of Public Policy*, London, Kogan Page/Tudor.

Sibeon, R. (1999) 'Anti-Reductionist Sociology', *Sociology*, 33(2).

Smith, A. and Russell, J. (1991) 'Using Critical Incidents in Nurse Education', *Nurse Education Today*, 11.

Smith, A. and Russell, J. (1993) 'Using Critical Incidents to Promote Reflection in Student Nurses', paper presented at the Reflective Learning and Reflective Practice Conference, University College North Wales.

Smith, M.J. (1998) *Social Science in Question*, London, Sage.

Smith, P.B. (1980) *Group Process and Personal Change*, London, Harper and Row.

Squires, G. (1993) 'Education for Adults', in M. Thorpe, R. Edwards and A. Hanson (eds) *Culture and Processes of Adult Learning*, London, Routledge.

Stainton Rogers, W. and Stainton Rogers, R. (1992) *Stories of Childhood*, Brighton, Harvester.

Stevens, R. (1983) *Freud and Psychoanalysis*, Milton Keynes, Open University Press.

Stretch, J.J. (1967) 'Existentialism: A Proposed Philosophical Orientation for Social Work', *Social Work*, 12(4).

Susser, M. (1968) *Community Psychiatry: Epidemiologic and Social Themes*, New York, Random House.

Taylor, I. (1996) 'Facilitating Reflective Learning', in N. Gould and I. Taylor (eds) *Reflective Learning for Social Work*, Aldershot, Arena.

Thomas, W.I. and Znaniecki, F. (1958) *The Polish Peasant in Europe and America*, New York, Dover.

Thompson, N. (1990a) 'More Than a Supervisor: The Developing Role of the Practice Teacher', *Journal of Training and Development*, 1(2).

Thompson, N. (1990b) 'The Uncertainty Principle in the Teaching of Social Work and Social Science', *Social Science Teacher*, 19(2).

Thompson, N. (1991a) 'The Practitioners' View: Gauging Perceptions in Social Work', *Social Science Teacher*, 21(1).

Thompson, N. (1991b) *Crisis Intervention Revisited*, Birmingham, Pepar.

Thompson, N. (1992a) *Existentialism and Social Work*, Aldershot, Avebury.

Thompson, N. (1992b) *Child Abuse: The Existential Dimension*, Norwich, University of East Anglia Social Work Monographs.

Thompson, N. (1995) *Age and Dignity: Working with Older People*, Aldershot, Arena.

Thompson, N. (1996) *People Skills: A Guide to Effective Practice in the Human Services*, London, Macmillan.

Thompson, N. (1997) *Anti-Discriminatory Practice*, 2nd edn, London, Macmillan.

Thompson, N. (1998a) *Promoting Equality: Challenging Discrimination and Oppression in the Human Services*, London, Macmillan.

Thompson, N. (1998b) 'The Ontology of Ageing', *British Journal of Social Work*, 28(5).

Thompson, N. (1998c) 'Towards a Theory of Emancipatory Practice', in B. Lesnik (ed.) *Countering Discrimination in Social Work*, Aldershot, Arena.

Thompson, N. and Bates, J. (1995) 'In-Service Training: Myth and Reality', *Curriculum*, 16(1).

Thompson, N. and Bates, J. (1996) *Learning from Other Disciplines: Lessons from Nurse Education and Management Development*, Norwich, University of East Anglia Social Work Monographs.

Thompson, N. and Bates, J. (1998) 'Avoiding Dangerous Practice', *Care: The Journal of Practice and Development*, 6(4).

Thompson, N., Murphy, M. and Stradling, S. (1994a) *Dealing with Stress*, London, Macmillan.

Thompson, N., Murphy, M. and Stradling, S. (1996a) *Meeting the Stress Challenge*, Lyme Regis, Russell House Publishing.

Thompson, N., Osada, M. and Anderson, B. (1994b) *Practice Teaching in Social Work: A Handbook*, 2nd edn, Birmingham, Pepar.

Thompson, N., Stradling, S., Murphy, M. and O'Neill, P. (1996b) 'Stress and Organizational Culture', *British Journal of Social Work*, 26(5).

Timms, N. (1968) *The Language of Social Casework*, London, Routledge and Kegan Paul.

Timms, N. and Timms, R. (1977) *Perspectives in Social Work*, London, Routledge and Kegan Paul.

Timms, N. and Watson, D. (1976) *Philosophy in Social Work*, London, Routledge and Kegan Paul.

Timms, N. and Watson, D. (1978) *Talking about Welfare: Readings in Philosophy and Social Policy*, London, Routledge and Kegan Paul.

Townsend, P. and Davidson, N. (1987) *Inequalities in Health*, Harmondsworth, Penguin.

UKCC (1986) *Project 2000: A New Preparation for Practice*, London, United Kingdom Central Council for Nursing, Midwifery and Health Visiting.

UKCC (1988) *Proposed Rules for the Standard, Kind and Content of Future Pre-Registration Nursing Education*, London, United Kingdom Central Council for Nursing, Midwifery and Health Visiting.

UKCC (1992) *Code of Professional Conduct*, London, United Kingdom Central Council for Nursing, Midwifery and Health Visiting.

Vince, R. (1996) *Managing Change: Reflections on Equality and Management Learning*, Bristol, The Policy Press.

Wilding, P. (1982) *Professional Power and Social Welfare*, London, Routledge and Kegan Paul.

Williams, F. (1989) *Social Policy: A Critical Introduction*, Cambridge, Polity.

Winch, P. (1958) *The Idea of Social Science and its Relations to Philosophy*, London, Routledge and Kegan Paul.

Wright, B. (1989) 'Critical Incidents', *Nursing Times*, 10 May.

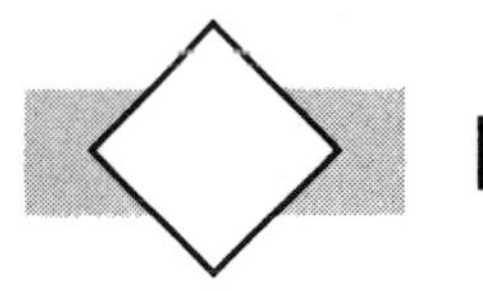

Index

Abbott, P., 55–6, 58, 60
Abercrombie, J., 125
abstract conceptualization, 5, 95
academic knowledge, 41
accountability, professional, 35
active experimentation, 6, 95
affirmation of diversity, 72
Agass, D., 8, 93–4
ageism, 11, 12, 74, 76, 126
analytical logic, 68–9
andragogy, 122
Andrisani, P.J., 115–16
anti-discriminatory practice, 10–14, 19, 31–2, 91, 92, 141
anti-intellectualism, 40, 85–6, 99–100, 141
applied research, 56–7
appraisal, 102
Argyris, C. and Schön, D.A., 22
Aron, R., 48
artistry, 66, 90, 96
authenticity, 77, 140

bad faith, 75–7, 140
Barnes, H., 75
Bate, P., 130–1
Bateson, G., 124
behaviourism, 27, 76, 120
Benner, P., 30
Benton, T., 37
bereavement, 35, 75
Berger, P., 25–6, 48–9, 70, 136
Best, S., 72
bias of theory, 36–8
Billington, R., 76–7
biology, 76
Black Report, 59
Boud, D.J., 6, 7, 94, 118, 126
Briggs Report, 111
Burr, V., 53

care of staff, 106–7
Carew, R., 110
Central Council for Education and Training in Social Work (CCETSW), 9, 16, 19, 114
challenge, and support, 106
child protection, 28, 34, 35, 56, 98, 139
children, in history, 36
Children Act 1989, 10, 55
Chinn, P.L., 21
class, 10, 14, 76, 126
clinical decisions, uncertainty and, 138
commitment, and professionalism, 9
'common sense' approach, 2, 13
  ideological nature of, 97–8
  inadequacy of, 31–2, 75
competence-based training, 118–21, 127, 143
Compton, B.R., 24–5
concrete experience, 5, 6, 95
concretization, 90
constructive alternativism, 135
continuous professional development (CPD), 34, 102–3, 133–5, 144
  IDP's overview, 134
  meta-learning as basis of, 124
  see also human resource development
control, locus of, 115, 116

Coutts-Jarman, J., 6–7, 30
Creasia, J.L., 8
creativity, 45, 98–9
Criminal Justice Act 1991, 10
crisis points, and professional intervention, 74–5
critical incident technique, 100–1
critical perspective, 111
critical theory, 52–3
cultural values, 14
culture
  organizational, 126, 128, 130–3
  and patterns of thinking, 137
  and sense of reality, 136
cultures, of academics and practitioners, 41
Curnock, K., 29, 32

data, interpretation of, 49
Davies, M., 110
debunking, 31
deductive research, 56
Department of Health, 35
dependency, ethos of, 12
depression, 12, 33, 74
Derrida, J., 71
determination, and influence, 76
determinism, 50
deutero-learning (meta-learning), 113, 124–6, 143
Dewey, J., 6–7
dialectical reason, 68–70, 79, 82, 142
  see also existentialism
différance, 71–2
Disabled People's Movement, 10
disablism, 13, 60, 76
discrimination, 10–14, 19, 31–2, 91, 92, 141
  and existentialism, 73
diversity, affirmation of, 72
Donald, J., 15
double hermeneutic, 50
Douglas, T., 94
Dunn, A., 17

eclecticism, 67, 87
education, 3, 54, 108, 109–10
  and knowledge, 112–13, 114, 118
  and self-knowledge, 117–18
  and skill development, 113–16, 118
  and training, 9, 110–12, 143
  and values, 116–17, 118
  see also learning; training
elitism, 9, 85, 99–100
empirical research, 44, 48–9
empowerment, ethos of, 12
enquiry and action learning (EAL), 105–6
Equal Opportunities Commission, 23
essentialism, 38
ethics, 17, 65
evaluation, 33–4
evaluative research, 57
Evans, D., 90, 124
Everitt, A., 18, 52–3, 60
  research-minded practice, 61–2, 98, 99
existentialism, 70, 72–3, 82–3
  authenticity, 77, 140, 142
  bad faith, 75–7, 140
  and dialectal interaction, 73, 82, 89–90
  existentialist practice, 80–1
  explanatory power of, 73
  lived experience, 79–80
  ontology, 73–7, 82
  phenomenology, 77–8, 88, 89
  and uncertainty, 138–40
experience
  hermeneutical science, 49
  HRD, 117, 118
  learning from, 5–7, 126
  lived, 79–80, 140
  phenomenology, 77–8
  subjective, 78
explanation, theory and, 22, 23
explanatory power, 58, 73
  validity and, 59, 65

fallacy of theoryless practice, 32–3, 96–7, 136
Feyerabend, P., 48
Field, J., 120–1
Fish, D., 81
fixed personality, 75–6
Fordism, 120–1
formal theory, 28–30
Foucault, M., 70
Fox, N.J., 71–2

fragmentation, 70–1
frameworks of thought, 15
frameworks of understanding, 22–5
freedom, responsibility and, 73, 75–7
Freire, P., 92
Further Education Unit, 95

Galaway, R.R., 24–5
Gambrill, E., 117, 138
Gardiner, T., 124–5
gender
  and adult learning, 122, 126
  awareness, 11
  see also sexism; women
Giddens, A., 45, 49, 50–1, 58
Gilbert, N., 57
Goddard, C., 110
Gould, N., 87–8
Gowin, D.B., 117
grand theories, 25, 26, 66
Griseri, P., 17
group approach, 101–2
groups, social, 52–3

Haber, J., 54
Habermas, J., 46, 58
Hall, S., 15
Hardiker, P., 29, 32
health
  and authenticity, 77
  positivism and, 46
  see also nursing
Heather, N., 44
'Heisenberg principle', 45
helplessness, learned, 130–1
hermeneutical science, 51–2, 53, 65
her story, 36
history, 36
Hollinger, R., 71
homeostasis, 74
Hopkins, J., 7
House, E., 138
Howe, D., 22, 33
Hughes, B., 12
Hugman, R., 9, 14
human resource development (HRD), 112, 127
  knowledge, skills and values, 127, 143
  see also education; person-centred learning; training
hypothesis formation, 5, 135, 136

identity, 73
ideographic theories, 26
ideology, 15–16, 137
  bias of theory, 36–8
imagination, sociological, 31
in-service training, 102
inappropriate responses, 35
individual, society and, 69–70
inductive research, 56
influence, and determination, 76
informal theory, 28–30, 32, 49
  integrating theory and practice, 96
information, and understanding, 49
informed practice, 1–2, 3, 14, 130–44
  and CPD, 133–5
  dealing with uncertainty, 138–40
  learning from experience, 6–7
  making it happen, 140–4
  organizational culture, 130–3
  practitioners as theorists, 135–8
  see also reflective practice
Institute of Personnel and Development (IPD), 134
integration of theory and practice, 90, 93–4
  optimizing, 140–4
  and professionalism, 9
  strategies for, listed, 94–107
interpretation of data, 49
interprofessional learning, 103
intervention, and crisis points, 74–5

jargon, 40
Johanssen, J., 130

Kellner, D., 72
Kellner, H., 25–6, 48–9
Kelly, G., 135–6, 144
knowledge
  academic, 40
  in action, 93
  gemeralized, 26
  in HRD, 112–13, 118, 127, 143
  within nursing practice, 30
  and power interests, 15

professionalism, 7–8, 9
research as source of, 17, 19, 54–5
self-, 117–18
knowledge bases
nursing, 7–8, 112, 113
social work, 114
'knowledge-in-action', 93
Knowles, M., 122
Kolb, D.A., 5–6, 95, 113, 124, 125
Kramer, M.K., 21

Laing, R.D., 51, 77, 81
language, 126
learned helplessness, 130–1
learning, 2, 109, 127, 140
and behaviour change, 95
continuous, 17
enquiry and action learning (EAL), 105–6
from experience, 5–7
interprofessional, 103
learner's responsibility for, 6, 7, 18, 125, 140
meaning in, 117, 120
'osmosis' approach, 89
'overlearning', 34, 97
person-centred, 122–6, 143
political context of, 91, 125–6
in practical context, 29
self-directed, 123, 143
spirit of, 119–20
see also continuous professional development; education; human resource development; training
learning cycle, 5–6, 95, 113
learning organizations, 132–3
learning sets, 101–2
Lecomte, R., 97
lived experience, 79–80, 140
LoBiondo-Wood, G., 54
locus of control, 115, 116
logocentrism, 71
Luckmann, T., 70, 136

Mahon, J., 80
meaning, 117, 120
Meleis, A.I., 124
mentoring, 104
meta-learning, 113, 124–6, 143
Mezirow, J., 91, 123
micro-theories, 25–6
middle-range theories, 25
Miles, R., 36
Mills, C.W., 31
models, theories and, 22–3
morale, 131
Mtezuka, M., 11
mystique of theory, 39–41, 86–7, 141

national vocational qualifications (NVQs), 118
nature, society and, 49
negative organizational culture, 130–1, 132
Nestel, I., 115–16
NHS and Community Care Act 1990, 10
nomothetic theories, 26
Novak, J.D., 117
nursing
and informal theory, 29, 30
knowledge base, 7–8, 112, 113
political context of, 16–17
professionalism, 9
rejection of routines, 34
and research, 18, 111

objectivity, 15, 25, 44, 45–6, 51, 58, 88
and dialectical reason, 69
Oliver, M., 13, 60
ontology, 73–7
oppression
anti-discriminatory practice, 10–14, 19, 31–2, 91, 92, 141
and bad faith, 76
and depression, 33
and existentialism, 73
research as source of, 60
organizational culture, 126, 128, 130–3
'overlearning', 34, 97

Page, G.T., 130
paradigms, 27
Parker, B., 8
Parse, R.R., 27
participative approach, 99

Pascall, G., 36–7
patriarchy, 23, 36–7
pedagogy, 122
person-centred learning, 122–6, 143
personal constructs, 135–6
personality, fixed, 75–6
perspective transformation, 91–2, 93
phenomenology, 77–8, 88, 89
philosophy, 2–3, 63–83, 142
dialectical reason, 68–70
eclecticism, 67
existentialism, *see* existentialism
postmodernism, *see* postmodernism
theory and, 64–7, 83
Pilalis, J., 32
political context, *see* sociopolitical context
positivism, 43–4, 59, 65, 140, 141
alternatives to, 50–7
critique of, 44–50
and research, 53–4
postmodernism, 53, 70–2
affirmation of diversity, 72
différance, 71–2
fragmentation, 70–1
logocentrism, 71
Powell, J.H., 34
power, 9, 14–15, 16, 37
practice
informed, 1–2, 14
theories of, 29–30
practice wisdom, *see* informal theory
practice-theory gap, *see* theory-practice gap
practice-theory integration, *see* integration of theory and practice
practitioners
and theorists, 40–1, 85
as theorists, 135–8, 144
'pragmatic' approach, *see* 'common sense' approach
praxis, 79
predetermination, 75
Preston-Shoot, M., 8, 93–4
Prior, L., 120
problem-setting/solving, 66
problematics, 22, 66
problematizing, 104–5
problems, and value judgements, 66
professional accountability, 35
professional development, continuous (CPD), 34, 102–3, 133–5, 144
IDP's overview, 134
meta-learning as basis of, 124
see also human resource development
professional intervention, and crisis points, 74–5
professional practice, and hermeneutical science, 52
professionalism, 1, 7–9, 18, 107, 141
Pugh, R., 53
pure research, 56–7

qualitative research, 56
quality circles, 101–2
quantitative research, 55–6

racism, 10, 11, 37, 76, 126, 137
Rafferty, D., 99–100
Ramazanoglu, C., 60
rationality, technical, 66, 78, 88, 121, 138, 140, 142
reality
existentialism and, 77–8, 79
personal/social construction of, 136
practitioners as theorists, 135–8
and social work practice, 40
reason
dialectical, 68–70, 79, 82, 142
see also existentialism
reductionism, 38
'reflection-in-action', 34, 88, 96
reflective observation, 5, 95
reflective practice, 3, 81, 85
CPD, 34
developing, 87–90
integration of theory and practice, 94–5, 107, 142–3
learning from experience, 6–7
organizational culture, 132
perspective transformation, 91–2
practitioners as theorists, 137–8
and research, 17
reification, 38–9
relevance-rigour dilemma, 65–6

reliability, of research, 58
religion, 76
research, 47, 53–61, 81–2, 141
  changing field, 59–60
  criteria, 57–8
  critical approach to, 18, 19
  education and, 111
  empirical, 44, 48–9
  limitations of, 59–60
  role of, 53–5
  social context, 47, 59
  as source of oppression, 60
  tentative nature, 59
  types of, 55–7
  value of, 17–18, 19
  see also research-minded practice
research stance, 58
research-minded practice, 60–2, 98–9
responses, inappropriate, 35
responsibility
  freedom and, 73, 75–7
  for learning, 6, 7, 18, 125, 140
rights, 16
rigour, 65–6, 98–9
  of research, 58
risk, 114, 139, 143–4
  see also uncertainty
Roberts, R., 24–5, 96
Roderick, C., 132–3
Rogers, C., 122–3
routines, rejection of, 34
Russell, J., 100

Sapey, B., 12
Sapsford, J.R., 55–6, 58, 60
Sartre, J.P., 69, 79
Schein, E.H., 130
Schön, D.A., 6, 91
  hermeneutical science, 52
  'knowledge-in-action', 93
  'overlearning', 34
  reflective practice, 88–9, 96
  relevance-rigour dilemma, 65–6
  research and professional practice, 98
  technical rationality, 66, 78, 88, 138
  theory/practice culture clash, 41
  uncertainty, 81
  see also Argyris, C. and Schön, D.A.
science, 2, 25, 43–53
  critical theory, 52–3
  critique of positivism, 44–50
  hermeneutical, 51–2
  see also research; social science
scientific thought, 42
scientism, 50, 51
Seaman, C.H.C., 54
self-awareness/knowledge, 117–18
self-directed learning, 123, 143
sexism, 10, 11, 12, 60, 93, 126
  and bad faith, 75, 76
  as marginalized issue, 37
  see also gender; women
sexual division of labour, 22–4, 36–7
Shipman, M., 58
Shotter, J., 49, 51, 61
Sibeon, R., 15, 28, 32, 40, 110
  evaluation of theories, 38–9
  on grand theories, 26–7
skills, 107–8
  HRD, 113–16, 118, 127, 143
Smith, A., 100
Smith, M.J., 48, 51, 53
social context
  existentialism, 76
  see also sociopolitical context
social groups, 52–3
social science
  changing field, 52
  distinctiveness, 49–50
  and positivism, 43, 44, 45
  and social context of research, 48
social work
  anti-intellectualism, 40
  classification of theory, 28–9
  education, 110, 111
  existentialism, 73, 77
  knowledge base, 7–8, 114
  positivism and, 46
  professionalism, 9
  research, 18
  sociopolitical context, 16
  values, 15–17
society
  individual and, 69–70
  nature and, 49
sociological imagination, 31

sociopolitical context
of learning, 91, 125–6
of nursing, 16–17
power, ideology and values, 14–17, 19
practitioners as theorists, 136–8
of research, 47, 48, 59
see also social context
Squires, G., 122
staff
care of, 106–7
morale, 131
Stainton Rogers, R., 36
Stainton Rogers, W., 36
stereotypes, 13
subjective experience, 78
subjectivity, 15, 51, 52, 88, 89
and dialectical reason, 69
supervision, 102
support, and challenge, 106
Susser, M., 87
'synthesis', 68–9

technical rationality, 66, 78, 88, 121, 138, 140, 142
teleology, 39
theories
evaluation of, 38–9
grand, 25, 26, 66
micro-, 25–6
middle-range, 25
and models, 22–3
of practice, 29–30
theorists
and practitioners, 40–1, 85
practitioners as, 135–8, 144
theory, 1, 2, 21–42
and anti-intellectualism, 40, 85–6, 99–100, 141
bias of, 36–8
costs of rejecting, 141
frameworks of understanding, 22–5
importance of, 30–6
mystique of, 39–41, 86–7, 141
not value-neutral, 19
person-centred learning, 123–4
and philosophy, 64–7, 83
in practice, 7
types and levels, 25–30
see also theories
theory-practice gap, 78, 84–108
developing reflective practice, 87–90
integrating theory and practice, 90, 93–4, 107
perspective transformation, 91–2
reasons for, 85–7
strategies for integration, listed, 94–107
theory-practice integration, *see* integration of theory and practice
theory-practice problematic, 15
theoryless practice, fallacy of, 32–3, 96–7, 136
Thomas, W.I., 78
Thompson, N., 32, 64–5, 115
anti-discriminatory practice, 10, 12
dialectal reason, 68
eclecticism, 67
existentialism, 74, 77, 79, 80
inadequacy of 'common sense', 31–2
informal theory, 29–30, 96
paradigms, 27
positivism, 45, 46
postmodernism, 53, 72
training and education, 110
uncertainty, 138, 139
Thompson, N. and Bates, J., 33
thought, frameworks of, 15
Timms, N., 32
totalization, 68, 69, 70
training, 3, 108, 109–10
competence-based, 118–21, 127, 143
and education, 9, 110–12, 143
in-service, 102
see also education; human resource development; learning
typifications, 136

UK Central Council for Nursing, Midwifery and Health Visiting (UKCC), 19, 113, 133
uncertainty, 81, 88, 142, 143–4
dealing with, 138–40
inevitability of, 45

understanding
  frameworks of, 22–5
  and information, 49
universal laws, 45

validity
  and explanatory power, 59, 65
  of research, 57
value judgements, and problems, 66
values, 15–17
  cultural, 14
  in HRD, 116, 118, 127, 143
  philosophy, 64–5
  science as value-free, 44, 46–8
  of theorists, 25
le vécu, 79, 80, 140
Vince, R., 89, 91

Walker, D., 94, 118, 126
Welfare State, 36–7
Weltanschauung, 25, 65, 117
Williams, F., 37
women
  and division of labour, 23, 24, 36–7
  see also gender; sexism
Wright, B., 100

SOCIAL POLICY
AN INTRODUCTION

Ken Blakemore

Social Policy: An Introduction is a comprehensive, readable and thought-provoking overview of current developments in social policy and welfare. It represents an ideal entry-point for students at degree and pre-degree level who are beginning studies in social policy. It also includes some in-depth discussion of key policy questions which will be of interest to professionals and practitioners in such fields as health, medicine and nursing, social services, education, law and policing.

This is the first introductory text in social policy to combine discussion of key policy-making themes (power and decision making, paying for welfare, social control, the role of the professions) with particular areas of social policy. There are separate chapters on social security, education, health, housing and environment, and community care, as well as on the history and principles of British social policy.

Readers will gain a perspective on the framework of social policy in Britain today, and also on why and how policies have developed in the way they have. In order to consolidate learning and to develop a critical approach, each chapter concludes with further questions and suggestions for research and reading. The book is completed with a glossary of key terms in social policy.

Contents

Preface – Acknowledgements – The subject of social policy – Ideas and concepts in social policy – The development of social policy in Britain – Who gets what? Slicing the welfare cake – Social policy and social control – who makes policy? The example of education – Are professionals good for you? Health policy and health professionals – Utopias and ideals; housing policy and the environment – Community and care – Conclusion: the future of social policy – Glossary – Bibliography – Index.

240pp 0 335 19493 1 (Paperback) 0 335 19494 X (Hardback)